MW01102564

The Silver Solution:
Ancient & Modern Secrets
for Health & Wellness

Bryan L Frank MD

The Silver Solution:
Ancient & Modern Secrets to Health & Wellness

Bryan L Frank MD, *Professional Association*
Re-Genesis Health: New Beginnings in Health & Wellness
PO Box 851952
Yukon, OK 73085-1952
www.TravelDoc.info

First published by Re-Genesis Health, July 2021.

ISBN: 978-0-578-94799-0

$20.00

ISBN 978-0-578-94799-0

52000>

9 780578 947990

Printed in Canada.

To order additional copies: Please visit www.TravelDoc.info.

Table of Contents

Praise for *The Silver Solution*

Infectious diseases are the most important consideration when traveling to many areas of the world and this book by Dr. Frank is a must have. Bryan has a vast 30+-year worldwide experience with essentially all types of infections. Our Canadian team has supplied silver to Dr. Frank and his charity, Global Mission Partners, Inc. for over a decade with incredible life-giving results to thousands of the disadvantaged worldwide. I have traveled to personally assist Bryan from early morning to late evening with frequently over 200 very ill patients a day. This hands-on true humanitarian is now providing us all, through this important book, the tools to travel safely and "pass it on".

- Dr. Brian Carpenter | *Natural Health Consultant, Developer of the new pH Structured Silver, Alberta, Canada*

Dr. Frank's book is organized in an easy manner for speedy application. I rely on silver as an important tool in my practice for prevention as well as resolving illness. Void of toxic side effects found in many current medicines, inexpensive silver is truly an ancient mineral which contributes to radically better health today.

- Trudy Pieper, ND | *author, "Prevention is the Cure for Cancer", cohost of American Christian Television Family & Friends health segments; 2014 ANMA Higher Achievement Award*

Dr. Frank has managed to write a thorough reference guide for practitioners and patients alike! His vast knowledge, understanding and practical application of silver is shown throughout the text of this book.

Silver is used more and more frequently in my office. In fact, our running joke for any ailment is, "put some silver on it." Although we laugh about it, it is undoubtedly true. Silver is an "anti-anything that shouldn't be in your body" solution. I, myself, have many testimonies to the effects of silver from treating EBV to common viral issues along with countless client testimonials. With the introduction of novel viruses in today's world I recommend everyone have silver on hand. It's a simple solution to modern ailments.

Blessings Abound,

- McKenzie Taylor ND CHS | *Naturopathic Doctor, Certified Health Specialist*

For all orphanages, international charitable organizations, business travelers or vacation travelers and long or short-term missionaries, I strongly recommend reading and taking this book, *The Silver Solution,* and his previous book, *Travel Well, Naturally,* on travel. Silver has dramatically changed life in my community. On a personal level I have been cured of malaria with silver sol treatment and I suffered a staph infection in my foot that was healed by the silver gel.

The Maisha Project has been using silver to support the health of over 900 orphans, 300 of which are students in our Maisha Academy, and 200 widows in Kenya for ten years. Dr. Bryan Frank has traveled to Maisha Orphanage in Kenya for the past 15 years and we have used silver for prophylaxis to prevent or to treat malaria, typhoid, dysentery and other infectious diseases that can easily strike one on travel in a challenging environment. I am personally anemic, and I take silver to help boost my immune system during my travel.

Join Dr. Bryan and a Global Mission Partners project to serve with us in Kenya! You will be warmly welcomed, and it may be the best travel of your life.

- Beatrice Williamson | *Founder, The Maisha Project, Kenya and Oklahoma City, OK*

Dr. Bryan Frank outlines methods and remedies that will aid people with nearly any health issue. As a Financial Writer, I end every issue with, "Wishing you health above wealth, wisdom beyond knowledge". This book is about making and keeping you healthy. As the ancients knew, when you have good health you are richer than any king. Dr. Bryan Frank, thank you for this impressive contribution to humanity.

- David Morgan | *Founder, TheMorganReport.com*

You may not know it yet, but silver occupies a unique and very important place in your life and for Medicine. Non-toxic Silver ions act as a fantastic catalyst, absorbing oxygen, and produces an antibiotic property. Silver has had an essential role in industry medicine for thousands of years. More recently, from the 1900s Dr. A.C. Barnes Argyrol to Silver sulfadiazine creams used for burns, silver and silver-protein complexes have been ingested or applied topically to fight illness.

You have in your hand a wonderful book - written by a preeminent exemplary Integrative Medicine and missionary physician. Dr. Frank gives you the secrets of silver and why you need it in your life. Read it. Digest it. It just may save your life!

- Robert D Milne MD | *Board Certified Family Practice, Integrative Medicine, Inventor of MVT-PCA pain therapy devices, Peace Corps, Paraguay 1970-73.*

About the Author

Bryan L Frank, MD is an integrative medicine physician from Oklahoma, an ordained pastor and missionary, and has coordinated and lead over 100 medical missions worldwide. Dr. Frank is President of ReGenesis Health, his private clinic, and of Global Mission Partners, Inc., a 501-c-3 Not-for-Profit Charitable Corporation.

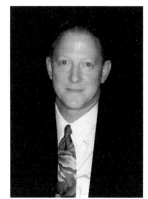

Dr. Frank is Board Certified in Integrative Pain Management, Medical Acupuncture and Anti-Aging & Regenerative Medicine and certified in Biomagnetic Pair and Advanced Bioenergetics therapies. He has authored numerous professional articles, chapters, books and atlases on medical acupuncture, Auricular Therapy, prolotherapy, neural therapy, integrative pain management and travel medicine.

Dr. Frank has led medical delegations to Russia, China, Korea and Japan for exchanging medical research and clinical expertise in medical acupuncture and other integrative, natural pain therapies. He has lectured internationally to medical congresses, symposia and seminars to many thousands of physicians and other healthcare workers in Europe, Asia, Oceana and North and South America. He served as President of the American Academy of Medical Acupuncture/AAMA (1999-2001) and as President of the International Council of Medical Acupuncture and Related Techniques/ICMART (2004-2006) and also as Vice-President of ICMART (2002-2004 and 2010-2012). He is Chief Medical Officer of UltraBotanica, LLC, maker of premium ultra-bioavailable botanical therapies.

As President of Global Mission Partners, Inc. (GMP), a 501-c-3 Not-for-Profit charitable corporation that serves the poor in developing parts of Asia, Africa, South America and North America, he has used silver, activated charcoal, botanical/herbal, homeopathic and essential oil natural therapies for maintaining health and/or treating a wide variety of medical conditions around the world. He has travelled to more than 60 countries on 6 continents through teaching, trekking and with his Mission teams. GMP currently serves Nepal, Kenya and México. He has 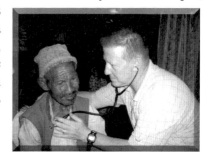 previously served in Russia, Costa Rica, Dominican Republic, Ecuador, India Haiti, Appalachia and Native American reservations. Information on GMP activities and opportunities for service may be found at www.GlobalMissionPartners.org.

Dr. Frank has led hundreds of volunteers over the last 30 years to serve tens of thousands of needy children and adults in over 100 missions for healthcare, construction, street children and orphan projects, water wells, community development, women's skills development, education, as well as preaching, teaching and Christian discipleship. He has travelled with his teams tackling malaria, Typhoid fever, leprotic infections, food poisoning, dysentery, and also common ailments such as coughs, colds, flu and various pain problems.

Dr. Frank has extensive travel and trekking experience, treating team members while on treks in the Himalaya, below the Matterhorn, Mt. Blanc and Machu Picchu, or while in bustling cities and tiny oxcart villages of Asia, Africa and Latin America as a global missionary. He has authored the Chapter, Principles of Pain Management in the renowned and definitive text, *Wilderness Medicine, 4th and 5th Editions*, and co-authored the Chapter, Medical Ethnobotany in *Wilderness Medicine, 7th Edition,* edited by the highly acclaimed Stanford Emergency Physician, Dr. Paul Auerbach.

Dr. Frank has also written numerous articles on Integrative Medicine, Medical Acupuncture, Prolotherapy, Neural Therapy, and other related techniques and has written and published the highly acclaimed text, *Auricular Medicine and Auricular Therapy: A Practical Approach, Atlas of Auricular Therapy and Auricular Medicine* and reference charts for Auricular Therapy and Hand Therapy, available at www.AuricularTherapy.com. He published the very helpful *Travel Well, Naturally: An essential guide to staying healthy on business, personal or mission travel,* showing people how to stay healthy naturally while on travel, or while staying home! See www.TravelDoc.info for information.

infection.pain.wound healing.burns.Ebola.malaria.dysentery
hepatitis.diarrhea.food poisoning.skin rash.Dengue Fever
Lyme's Disease.sunburn.sea sickness.MRSA.sepsis.anthrax
cough.cold.flu.bronchitis.superbugs.gastroenteritis.typhoid

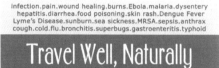

Travel Well, Naturally

An Essential Guide to Staying Healthy on Personal, Business or Mission Travel

Bryan L. Frank, M.D.

strep throat.trauma.bacteria.viruses.fungus.parasites.HIV
drug resistant infections.herpes.shingles.pink eye.jet lag
stings.bites.tooth abscess.UTI.hangover.heat stroke.cholera
vomiting.intestinal worms.accidents.pain.otitis.pharyngitis

Travel Well, Naturally guides the domestic or international traveler to stay healthy or get well naturally. Author Dr. Bryan L. Frank has traveled to over 60 countries, with over 100 missions and teaching tours on 6 continents for over 30 years. His teams are effectively tackling malaria, food poisoning, dysentery, cholera, hepatitis and also common ailments such as coughs, colds, flu and various pains. He provides practical, easy-to-reference tables and illustrations for using the new Structured Silver, activated charcoal, botanical or herbal remedies, homeopathic remedies and essential oils to prevent or recover from scores of travel illnesses, plus a separate chapter on natural pain management for travel.

Specializing in Anesthesiology, Medical Acupuncture, Natural Pain and Sports Medicine and Anti-Aging & Regenerative Medicine, Dr. Frank has a unique ability to share health and wellness from a truly integrative paradigm. You should travel well and healthy with *Travel Well, Naturally*.

"*Travel Well, Naturally* is surely a tool any intrepid traveler could and should pack in their travel kit"
Pamela W. Smith, MD, MPH, MS
Director, A4M Fellowship in Metabolic, Nutritional and Functional Medicine

"...this handbook details natural therapeutic gems that every traveler should carry and use when needed on their worldwide journeys."
Robert D. Milne, MD, Inventor of MVT-PCA pain therapy devices,
Peace Corps, Paraguay 1970-1973

"After more than 2 million miles traveling to some of the most remote places in the world, I can think of so many times I wish I had this powerful knowledge for myself and those who traveled with me.
Steve Whetstone, Senior VP International Operations, Feed the Children 1998-2014

"*Travel Well, Naturally* is a must read for travelers in today's world of infections diseases. It is truly a message of hope and love."
Gordon Pedersen, PhD, ND, Immunologist, Toxicologist, Olympic Medalist, Best Selling Author

Travel Well, Naturally, travel health products and information are available at www.TravelDoc.info

Disclaimer

Integrative and alternative (non-conventional) health therapies and even conventional medical practices, are constantly changing through the development of researchers and practitioners worldwide. *The Silver Solution* presents information felt by this author to be current and relative at the time of writing, though it is expected that additional and different insights and understandings will be appreciated in time. The information in this guide is not intended to diagnose, treat, cure or prevent disease, as these skills may only be practiced by appropriate licensed healthcare providers.

Readers are advised to confirm that information regarding diagnosis, prevention, treatment, self-treatment and healthcare practitioners they are seeking is current, valid, appropriate and that it complies with the legislation and practice standards applicable to the given situation.

This book is not intended to replace sound medical advice. It is intended to present options for maintaining or regaining health and wellness. *Always consult a physician or health care provider when you are in need.* All patients are advised to seek the consultation of competent and informed licensed health care providers. This author and the publisher are not responsible for any adverse effects or consequences arising from the use or misuse of any of the material presented or omitted.

THE FDA HAS REVIEWED NONE OF THE STATEMENTS IN THIS BOOK. *Consult your personal healthcare provider before beginning or changing any therapeutic supplemental or prescription regimen.*

As this writing is designed to be easy to read for the lay public, the book is not footnoted within the body of the text, by design. A strong set of references is given for those who wish to explore further resources, from those references used by the author and others as well.

What Experts Are Saying About Silver

"Silver solutions have presented in both basic research and clinical experience as remarkable therapeutics in many diverse clinical situations. Research on silver demonstrates antibacterial, antiviral, antifungal and antiparasitic effects for virtually every surface and tissue of the body. Silver is both highly effective clinically and is without toxicity. These properties make silver a preferred therapeutic for treating patients, healthcare volunteers and team members in international missions and humanitarian efforts."

- Dr. Bryan Frank, MD | President, Global Mission Partners, Inc.
President, Re-Genesis Health: New Beginnings in
Health & Wellness

"Few things in life are as cut-and-dried as the fact that silver is completely safe when used within normal limits."

- Dr. Herbert Slavin, MD | Director, Institute of
Advanced Medicine in Lauderhill Florida

"Anything in excess has consequences. Common substances like table salt and aspirin are harmless with normal use, but excessive intake can become toxic and even life-threatening. With normal responsible usage, silver supplements are entirely harmless to humans."

- Dr. Jeffrey Blumer, MD, PhD | Former Director of the
Center for Drug Research

"Over the past few years, several new studies have demonstrated the fact that silver is one of the most effective agents in the battle against MRSA and other deadly antibiotic-resistant super pathogens..."

- Dr. Joseph Mercola, DO | Best-Selling Author

"Over time, the well-established indications for the effective use of silver were for water purification, wound dressings for the promotion of healing, the prevention and treatment of infection, dental hygiene ... eye conditions ... and other infectious conditions."

- Dr. J. Wesley Alexander, MD, Sc.D. | Professor Emeritus of Surgery, University of Cincinnati

"Not a day goes by without one of my patients informing me of another miraculous experience with structured silver. I use it extensively in my practice for multiple infective and inflammatory conditions. Absolutely indispensable for me and my patients"

- Dr. Trethart, MD | Clinical Physician

"What is the future? The new vectors for designing water-based products for use in major industries and for maintaining health or causing healing are just legion now. [...] The sky is the limit. [...] Structuring of water by colloidal silver or by radiation now becomes possible for the human race, and we think it is the most benign, easiest vector to use for many, many processes."

- Dr. Rustum Roy, PhD | Professor, Pennsylvania State University

"As I am trying to change the way all autoimmune diseases (ADs) are treated worldwide, pH Structured Silver solution is vital in addressing the chronic, stubborn infections that are always involved. When working to reverse and prevent all AD, rather than just using a band-aid medicine to address the symptoms in only one body part, addressing the causes of the AD must happen. Being able to treat all the different types of infections involved in every patient with the pH Structured Silver is a game changer. Whether the infections are viral, fungal, bacterial, parasitic, tick-borne or mycoplasma, this product can clear them all at the same time. Patients appreciate the easy dosing schedule and the ability to use it for as many months, or longer, as needed to clear the infections and reverse their autoimmune diseases."

-David Bilstrom, MD | Director of the International Autoimmune Institute & Bingham Memorial Center for Functional Medicine

Preface

The world we live in is vastly different than prior to the Industrial Revolution. Previously, people understood where food came from and how it was raised. We were able to depend on our doctors to have our health prevention or recovery as their main priority. While many physicians are sincere in their efforts to care for their patients, medical education and pharmaceutical marketing has led to an overall shift in focus from healthcare to disease management. This shift can be easily noticed in three industries of our society: Agriculture, Food and Medicines or Pharmaceuticals.

Agriculture

Despite the evident and complex links between health, nutrition and agriculture, money, not improving health, is a more prevalent goal of agriculture policy. Time is money, product is money, and cutting cost is saving money. Large-scale farming or "industrial farms" rely on cutting costs to produce great quantities of more profitable foods, often at the expense of our health.

Factory farm characteristics include:
- Dominating the industry, especially the meat industry.
- Raising animals in economical but large, cramped and unhealthy facilities and unnatural foodstuff.
- Preventing illnesses from these cramped conditions by raising animals on antibiotics.
- Growing crops that are genetically modified to produce bigger, bug-resistant and environmentally resistant crops, but which may confer toxicity once ingested.
- Overuse of pesticides, herbicides and fertilizers and to strip the land of vital nutrients and minerals.

The food we take home from our local and superstore markets may very likely be harming our families daily. Thus, agricultural changes have led to the next industry danger, food.

Food

Food was once understood as a source of sustenance and pleasure yet today our dinner tables can be a minefield. We actually do not even know *what* we are eating commonly. What appears to be good ground hamburger meat may actually be a bit of meat with a whole lot of fillers, chemicals and other harmful substances. There is currently a move to encourage synthetic "meats". The yogurt we love so much and is advertised as 'high in protein' may actually be filled with genetically modified soy derivatives which increase the 'protein' percentage but contain high levels of physic acid, an anti-nutrient that robs important vitamins and minerals from the body, as well as glyphosate (Round Up®), which is used in farming practices in much of America today.

Some alarming facts about food:
- More than two-thirds of adults and nearly one-third of youth are clinically overweight or obese.
- More evidence is showing that the types of food we eat have a worsening effect on our gut health and immune system.
- The Standard American Diet (SAD!) consists of foods loaded with saturated fats, refined sugars, food colorings, artificial sweeteners and toxins from agricultural practices.
- Many foods, often even fresh fruits and vegetables, are processed, thus losing their natural benefits.

Regularly consuming these "pseudo-foods" may lead to significant health problems, thus many often turn to the next industry danger, Medicines and Pharmaceuticals.

Medicines or Pharmaceuticals

The physician-patient relationship, much like that with our pastors or faith leaders, is sacredly personal and bound by accepted norms of practice. Patients rely on their healthcare providers to help them make life-saving decisions. Physicians, in turn, depend on patients to be honest in order to offer the highest quality medical advice. While likely most or all physicians seek to offer the best health advice, medical education and continuing medical education, as well as the promotion of patented pharmaceuticals through their representatives, has led to many physicians being trained to believe that the only or the best solution for health problems are in the latest patented pharmaceutical medicine.

Further, many physicians are totally ignorant that many natural therapies provide health benefits as good or even better than what they learned in medical training or from the "drug rep" over a free lunch, while many of the natural therapeutics are void of toxic side effects so prevalent with many patented medications.

Concerns about Medicines or Pharmaceuticals:
- Pharmaceutical companies only develop patented drugs if there is a large profit to be made.
- Pharmaceuticals generally treat the symptoms and seldom cure people, as patients would no longer need the drug and therefore the profits would be greatly limited.
- Pharmaceutical drug prices are high and continue to increase.
- The medical industry is not sustainable in its present dependence on patented pharmaceuticals.
- Many doctors are taught, even threatened if not compliant, to prescribe pharmaceuticals to cover the symptoms rather than treat the root of the problem, often with natural solutions.

Many patients thus feel like they are in a no-win situation. Their physicians may be caring and kind but without education to understand safe and effective options, their only tool is often the massively powerful pharmaceutical industry or Big Pharma. While much of our food is often poisoning us or, at best, not nourishing us with essential vitamins, minerals and other nutrients, the medications we commonly take are not even designed to heal but only to manage our sickness and diseases.

Taking Back Control

This book is not about politics but through the political we can control what happens in our society. Voting for someone who is informed of the many alternatives to health, agriculture and nutrition, and the proper role of pharmaceuticals, and who understands and speaks to our needs and concerns is critical to turn our society back to a more sensible time where policies and practices will again be supporting health and wellness rather than managing disease.

Fortunately, there is a growing organic food industry in the USA where GMO seed and chemical fertilizers, pesticides and such are avoided. When possible, choose organic produce and organic farm raised grass-finished meats, and buy locally from farmer's markets. Supporting the smaller, local farmers will provide us meals with the nutrients that help our bodies maintain or regain health.

I want you to heal and to prosper, and I want to see you go and help others to heal and prosper as well. However, we cannot help someone else until we have helped ourselves, so let us explore healing ourselves.

Key Takeaway: Preface

- Agriculture, food and medicine are taking a toll on your health.
- Agriculture focuses on mass production by large-scale farming.
- This causes an overuse of antibiotics, pesticides and fertilizers.
- Our food is not as nutritious as in prior eras.
- Significant portions of our population are greatly overweight.
- Much of our food is destroying our gut health and immune system.
- Most of our food is processed.
- Medication is often managing disease, not healing you.
- Pharmaceutical companies are focused on money, not your health.
- Drug prices are high and still climbing.
- You need to vote and wisely use your purchasing power to change society.
- Advocate for your health and your family.

Chapter I

You Are Designed for Healing

It is remarkable that despite our food being stripped of nutrition and our medicines often making us sicker, we still survive. How can that be? Our bodies are in a dynamic state, protected by many remarkable defense mechanisms that are constantly functioning behind the scenes from the moment that you were born until your death. These health defense systems protect us and keep our cells and our organs and tissues functioning properly. Some of these systems are so powerful that they can even reverse diseases like cancer and although these systems work independently, they also support and interact with one another.

You are a healing machine

As Dr. William Li, author of *Eat to Beat Disease* explains, "[There are] five defense systems which form key pillars to your health. These five different systems are *angiogenesis, regeneration, [gut] microbiome, DNA protection,* and *immunity*".

- *Angiogenesis* is the formation of blood vessels. There are over 60,000 miles of blood vessels that course throughout our bodies and bring oxygen and nutrients to all your cells, tissues and organs.
- *Regeneration* is largely accomplished by our body's stem cells. With more than 750,000 stem cells distributed throughout your bone marrow, lungs, liver and almost all of your organs, your body has the ability to regenerate itself every day. The stem cells maintain, repair and regenerate your body throughout your entire life.
- *Gut microbiome* is the most important microbiome in our bodies. Approximately 40 trillion bacteria inhabit our bodies, most of which act to defend our health. Not only do these bacteria produce health supporting metabolites from the

foods we ingest and deliver it to our gut, they also can control our immune systems, influence angiogenesis and even help produce hormones that influence our brain and social function. Specifically, up to 90% of serotonin, the "happy hormone", is made in our gut!

- *DNA* is the genetic blueprint which our bodies use to develop you when we were in our mother's womb. It also is the blueprint for every single cell in our body, except blood cells, when cells replicate. Our DNA is also designed as a defense system. As such, many repair mechanisms that protect us against damage caused by solar radiation, household chemicals, stress, compromised sleep and poor diet, are regulated by our DNA.

- *Immunity* defends our health in very sophisticated and advanced ways. It is influenced by our gut and is one of these main reasons that we are not sick every time we leave our house.

These five pillars make up our natural foundation for fighting disease. Each has its own function and contributes to our health, and they work in synchrony to ensure we can maintain our jobs, play with our kids and give our pets big kisses. But at times, one of the pillars becomes damaged and ineffective.

What went wrong?

Our bodies are usually quite effective at managing the stresses and pollutants that we encounter every day. For example, we may eat a tuna sandwich for lunch every day, and normally our body is able to deal with the trace amounts of mercury and expel it. However, at some point we may find that instead of being removed, the mercury is accumulating and attacking our thyroid. This may trigger an autoimmune disease called Hashimoto's Thyroiditis. Or, perhaps we always enjoyed eating all types of foods, but now favorite meals like eggs or ice cream make us incredibly ill. These kinds of ailments can really startle someone who has never really given their health much thought.

So, what can be done to stop the damage that is affecting our body?

What does health mean? To most people, health is the absence of disease. To mainstream medicine, it is assumed that a patient who is free of disease symptoms is more or less healthy and the aim for pharmaceuticals is to achieve this condition by removing any disagreeable symptoms. In holistic or natural medicine, health is regarded not just as an absence of disease symptoms, but as a state of profound physical, emotional and mental wellbeing so that we cannot develop a disease. Consideration of health and wellbeing is a critical understanding for us to live well.

If we desire to maintain or pursue outstanding health, we must work for it by consciously minimizing the multitude of negative influences on our health and maximize positive influences instead. Constantine Hering's Law of Cure is the basis of all healing, or the law of the direction of symptoms, and states that *"From above downwards. From within outwards. From a more important organ to a less important one. In the reverse order of their coming."*. He suggests that symptoms of a chronic disease disappear in a definite order, going in reverse order of their appearance and taking about a month for every year the symptoms have been present. Symptoms move from the more vital organs to the less vital organs (for complete regeneration); from the interior of the body towards the skin and finally, symptoms move from the top of the body downward.

As Hippocrates once said, "All disease begins in the gut", and although he said this statement centuries ago, it still stands valid today. It's estimated that approximately 70-80% or more of chronic diseases stem from a disorder within the gut, due to the importance the gut plays in our immune system. The gut protects us from infection, supports metabolism and promotes the two keys to cellular health - absorption of nutrients and the elimination of toxins. This being said, it is critical to heal the gut in order to maintain or regain physical and mental health and wellness.

Your go-to solution

Silver solutions, gels and drops may be your greatest secrets to promote health and wellness. These likely should be our go-to tools to combat many of life's ailments. Silver may greatly assist in healing the gut (and many more things) and supporting the immune system on many levels. The newest silver products are comprised of pH-balanced, structured (energized), nano-particle silver ions held in aqueous solution.

In 2009, the American Chemical Society found that silver nanoparticles are safer and much more effective than previous silver products, such as silver salts, silver proteins or ionic silver solutions. An additional advantage of the structured silver solutions is that bacterial resistance does not occur. Silver solutions and gels should be readily available in our first aid kits, make-up bag and nutritional shelf.

Key Takeaway: You Are Designed for Healing!

- There are five defense systems which form key pillars to your health.
- *Angiogenesis* is the formation of blood vessels.
- *Regeneration* by stem cells maintain and repair our body throughout life.
- The *gut microbiome* is the most important microbiome due to its role in immunity and metabolite production.
- *DNA* is your genetic blueprint which makes you, you.
- *Immunity* defends your health in impressive and complex ways.
- Our bodies can be overwhelmed by pollutants and toxins.
- Structured silver solutions and gels should be leading tools in our First Aid Kit.

Chapter 2

Introduction to Silver

What is silver?

Silver is one of the most important metals a person can obtain, not because of its monetary value in global supply, or its current "price" or investor sentiment, nor because it makes a nice set of earrings or tableware. Silver is one of the most important metals because silver is perhaps nature's finest germ killer. Silver's elemental properties are toxic to pathogenic microorganisms while simultaneously being non-toxic to healthy cells and probiotic bacteria. This is an outstanding discovery that changed the way humans looked at healing with silver. Silver is today where penicillin was 80 years ago, but silver is not burdened with penicillin's negative attributes, and we do not need a prescription to utilize silver to care for our families.

Silver throughout history

Silver has a fascinating role throughout history to become the amazing therapeutic it is today. Ancient Greeks in the 9th century BC used silver vessels to purify their water before consumption. Looking forward from then several thousand years, American pioneers trekking westward in the 1860's used silver to keep their water safe and prevent dysentery, colds and flu. To this day, people in India still wrap some food and candies in a thin silver foil to prevent spoilage, which is typically consumed with the food. Business India estimates that an astonishing 275 tons of silver foil is eaten annually in India.

Some have heard the expression of 'being born with a silver spoon in [their] mouth' and think that this expression refers to one's status, which is partly true, but the analogy goes much deeper than that. When children used to get sick, they were told to suck on a silver spoon (only the wealthy had actual silver tableware, hence the connotation that the analogy is about wealth) in order to prevent an illness from progressing. The saying is not about showing off wealth, rather about silver's ability to stop infections. Some of the silver utensils enjoyed by the wealthy were of poor quality, however, and could lead to a blueish pigmentation after long-term use, hence the term for these wealthy as "blue bloods".

Research demonstrating silver's ability to control infections, even those of antibiotic-resistant super infections, is truly impressive. In the 1980's, Dr. Ford from UCLA Medical School documented over 650 different disease-causing pathogens that were destroyed in minutes when exposed to trace amounts of silver. Unlike its modern prescription antibiotic counterpart, silver does not lead to resistance or immunity in the bacteria that are killed by it. This is a major advantage for our health as the Center for Disease Control and Prevention (CDC) reported that more than 2.8 million people in the U.S. suffer illnesses every year as a result of antibiotic-resistant infections and sadly 35,000 people die from these infections.

People have known silver's benefits for fighting infections for thousands of years and many silver products, ancient and new, have come from this characteristic. Medicinal silver compounds were developed in the late 1800s and many patients enjoyed widespread use of silver compounds, salves and colloidal solutions prior to 1930. By 1940, there were approximately 48 different silver compounds marketed and used to treat virtually every infectious disease in America. These silver compounds were available in oral, injectable and topical forms.

Since 1973, silver has been shown in research to have topical activity against 22 bacterial species (643 isolates) including gram-positive and Gram-negative bacteria (6 isolates). Ongoing investigations into the effect of and properties of silver continues around the world today. New advances continue in the pursuit of maximum silver solution effectiveness and safety. In just the past few years, new methods of structuring silver molecules into water have been developed that show significant improvements when compared with earlier colloidal and hydrosol silver solutions.

Structured silver is a new, critical distinction

Critically important, structured silver is not the same as other silver products. All other products that contain silver and water are not the same as structured silver solutions.

One thousand years ago, people used primitive forms of silver and received some anti-microbial benefits. One hundred years ago, people use primitive colloidal and ionic silver products and receive good antimicrobial benefits, but also, at times, suffered side effects of argyria, a blueish-gray discoloration of the skin which is rare and non-life-threatening. Argyria can occur with concentrated silvers (solutions with a very high ppm/parts per million) and impure silver compounds (eg. silver salts) that precipitate within the body. Argyria does not occur with advanced structured silver solutions when it is taken as suggested because the silver nanoparticles do not collect in the body. Ten years ago, people used more advanced silver solutions, hydrosols and gels, and received excellent antimicrobial benefits and vastly improved safety standards.

When choosing your silver products, one may not be able to see the difference with the naked eye, but there are real differences that can impact your health. Home-made and even some store-bought silver solutions may not be as safe or as effective as the newest generation of pH balanced, structured silver solutions.

Unfortunately, many medical experts remain unaware of the interrelationships between physics, energy, healing and silver. When questioned about silver, many experts still respond in terms of biochemistry, a decades-old approach suitable for decades-old silver solutions that worked through biochemistry. However, the biochemical paradigm is insufficient for understanding and applying today's advanced silvers, which are built on a biophysics model. A rapidly growing number of doctors are making use of the latest silver technologies, but many more doctors still think in an obsolete paradigm. This is an unfortunate shortcoming of today's medical field in its lack of understanding of advancements in silver solutions.

Structure and Composition

In order to better understand how structured silver products differ from older silver products, two terms need to be understood: structure and composition.

As methods of making and using silver have advanced over the centuries, the primary focus has been on chemistry. But the properties of effective silver do not stop with chemistry. Newer forms of silver also use physics to further improve their applications. There are several products on the market with excellent chemistry, but very few with excellent physics. The difference in performance is demonstrated in lab results and clinical healing times, but many people are not yet accustomed to thinking in terms of biophysics and thus find the difference a bit confusing.

Composition refers to the ingredients of a substance while structure refers to the way that those ingredients are arranged. Two quick examples that will demonstrate the differences in meaning:

1. Graphite, coal and diamonds have identical ingredients. They are all composed of 100% carbon. The significant difference is the way the carbon molecules are arranged. Search the internet for "graphite vs diamond" to see that structural differences create such radically different properties!

2. Similarly, consider a box of Lego toys. If you gave 100 Lego pieces to a dozen children, you would soon see a dozen different structures pieced together. Despite having identical composition, different children would each make different structures: one would make a tower, one a house, one a spaceship, etc.

Structure and composition are related but are not the same. Newcomers to medicinal silver see several silver products on the market that contains similar ingredients and conclude that these products must all be the same. However, structural differences create significant and important differences in properties.

There are many different types of silver products, but for the most part there are only three that make up the majority of silver products available on the market today. Those are structured nano-silver products, ionic silver products and silver protein products. While some types of silver products are useful, others may not be very effective, or even safe at all. Most silver products will eventually kill some bacteria and other pathogens if given a long enough period of time and if they contain a high enough concentration of silver to do so.

Ionic silver products

Ionic silver products work because each silver ion is missing one electron, which means it has a positive charge. The silver ion wants the electron back, so it will steal an electron from the cell wall of a bacteria, for example. When it steals the electron from the cell wall of a bacteria, it creates a hole in the bacterial cell membrane. If enough silver ions poke enough holes in the bacterial cell membrane, the bacteria die.

Summary of Ionic Silver Products:
- Most common type of silver liquid found in the supplement industry.
- These often have small particle size, but often are the least stable and may easily fall out of suspension.
- Due to its mechanism of destroying pathogens, it is considered "*a one and done technology*".
- May be metabolized and in extreme cases (constant consumption of large doses over many years), the silver may build up in the body and cause argyria, also known as the Blue Man Syndrome.

These products are usually heavily marketed, overpriced and often with very little real product testing or information.

Silver protein solutions

Silver protein solutions commonly contain larger amounts of silver and thus they sometimes need to be bound to a protein to stay in suspension. Binding the ionic silver to a protein allows the silver to stay suspended in water for longer periods of time. However, as a result of binding with proteins, the silver ions are less functional or useful than traditional ionic silver ions.

Older nano silver products

Some older nano silver products on the market function much the same as ionic products. These older products are easy to identify because they are yellow to brown in color. While these products will probably function at some level, they still only have one mode of action. The new improved nano-silver products are clear in color and have multi-action capabilities.

Structured silver nanoparticle products

Critically, structured silver nano-products are not the same as other silver products. Even other products that contain silver and water are not the same.

Summary of structured silver nanoparticle products:
- They contain metallic nanoparticles of silver.
- These are the most stable form of silver solution.
- These solutions may remain stable for many years due to the high zeta potential.
- They may kill bacteria and other pathogens at very low levels of silver concentrations (very low ppm).

So, despite structured silver having, in some cases, identical ingredients as older or inferior silver products, the differences due to structure may be very significant.

pH-balanced, structured silver solution differences include:
- pH Structured Silver has an alkaline pH whereas older silver hydrosols are acidic.
- They have a low surface tension, as measured in dynes, leading to better absorption and utilization.
- They have magnetic properties.

- These solutions are currently the highest quality colloidal silvers.
- These solutions have resonant energy.
- These solutions demonstrate radically different structures which become visible when frozen (structured silver creates coherent macrostructures that are visible when in solid form, whereas older silvers and tap water create random crystal structures).

Importantly, the water in structured silvers is not just a carrier of silver. It is more than an inert solution. The water within structured silver has been structured or energized and acts as an important part of the molecular structure. Structured silver, due to this structure, has a lower surface tension which cells need to maximize absorption and cellular energy transfers.

For more information on the structures of water and their very important differences, read *Fourth Phase of Water* by Professor Gerald Pollock and other books on structured water in References.

So, what does silver really do?

In short, silver kills germs. Billions of germs (bacteria, viruses, fungi, parasites) that live anywhere on or in your body can be causing you illness, or pathogenic. Germs living in your pores may be causing acne, while those in the vagina may cause vaginal infections, those on the lips may be causing cold sores, and those in the digestive tract causing gas and many serious health problems. The possibilities are endless. If you can name a spot on or in your body and you can get silver into contact with germs that are growing there, silver solutions or gels can likely assist you to heal.

Which germs will silver affect?

Silver has been shown to be effective with multiple categories of pathogens, often outperforming conventional antibiotics, which typically have a limited spectrum of activity (they only kill a few specific microbes or germs) and in some cases, they kill the good microbes (probiotics) along with the bad microbes, which may be very harmful to our health.

Structured silver is a broad-spectrum antimicrobial that research has shown to:
- Destroy pathogenic bacteria.
- Inhibit viral replication (both DNA and RNA viruses).
- Destroy many fungi, yeasts and protozoa.
- Destroy numerous amounts of parasites (reports show decades of success with killing the malaria parasite in thousands of malaria-positive patients).

Silver has even been shown to kill antibiotic resistant strains of bacteria such as MRSA (Methicillin Resistant Staphylococcus Aureus). Antibiotic-resistance is a major problem facing hospitals, nursing care facilities and even homes today. As pathogenic bacteria no longer respond to antibiotics such as penicillin, methicillin, vancomycin and others, we are at greater risk of picking up a germ that we cannot kill with conventional pharmaceuticals.

However, silver kills bacteria differently than traditional antibiotics, which kill resistant and non-resistant bacteria alike. Pathogenic bacteria have a water-soluble cell membrane and therefore are susceptible to structured silver. "Good bacteria" have a lipid cell membrane like human cells and are not disturbed by the silver solutions. This may reflect an evolutionary symbiosis of helpful bacterial cells and human cells through evolutionary changes. This allows us to keep this secret weapon at home in our medicine cabinet and may help you protect our families when many various antibiotics cannot. Importantly, even with silvers ability to kill pathogens, it is safe to be used at home on a regular daily basis.

Key Takeaway: Introduction to Silver

- Silver's elemental properties are toxic to pathogenic micro-organisms while simultaneously being non-toxic to healthy cells and probiotic bacteria.
- Silver has been used in throughout history due to its anti-microbial properties.
- Medicinal silver compounds were widespread by the 1930's in the USA and some are still in use today.
- There are many different types of silver products, but they do not all work as effectively.
- Most common silver solutions are structured silver nano-products, ionic silver products, and silver protein products.
- Structure and composition are not the same and may produce very different characteristics.
- Structured silver is superior as it utilizes both biochemistry and biophysics.
- Structured silver kills resistant and non-resistant bacteria alike, unlike many conventional pharmaceutical antibiotics.

Chapter 3

Silver Safety

With the tremendous diverse benefits and many varied applications of silver solutions, one of the greatest aspects of using many silver products is its remarkable safety. The newer pH balanced, structured silver products are safe enough to be used at home on a regular daily basis, and no prescription or a hefty price tag is required as with patented pharmaceuticals.

Silver may be used safely internally or on any external surface or orifice, including the eyes, ears, nose, mouth, anus or vagina.

If taken internally, silver selectively kills pathogenic bacteria while leaving the healthy bacteria (probiotics) unharmed. The selective action on beneficial versus pathogenic bacteria is due to the beneficial bacteria's double layer of fatty (lipid) protection on the outside (similarly to our human cells), as opposed to the water-soluble cell membrane found in pathogenic bacteria. Further, this fatty layer protects probiotics from stomach acid, allowing them to grow and contribute to digestion. In the same manner, this fatty layer protects probiotics from the water-based silver's antimicrobial action.

Further safety considerations include:
- Silver is not considered to be a heavy metal according to Merck Manual of Diagnosis and Therapy and it cannot accumulate in the brain. Silver is the only metal that is not considered to be a heavy metal because it does not produce heavy metal poisoning.
- Silver is non-toxic at recommended dosages and 90-99% of ingested silver leaves the body unmetabolized within 24 hours.
- Silver is already being used in many places such as hospitals, space shuttles, washing machines, water filters and many other settings for its ability to control unwanted microbes and

to heal wounds such as burns, bed sores, diabetic ulcers and more.

Ingesting silver is normal

Some people may be concerned that ingestion of silver is not normal, however, most people ingest silver every day as silver is found in many foods. Mushrooms contain silver concentrations as high as several hundred parts per billion. Most meats contain silver and silver is even found in our drinking water, lakes and rivers. The World Health Organization estimates that people typically consume between 20 and 50 micrograms of silver on a daily basis.

Not surprisingly, silver is found in our bodily tissues. One of the highest concentrations of silver is within the platelets of our blood. This is interesting as platelets are an essential part of the body's natural healing response.

Although we encounter silver on a daily basis through our diets and environment, not all forms of silver are the same. Some forms of silver can be harmful, such as silver proteins, silver salts, and industrial byproducts containing silver. The newest pH balanced, structured silver is ultra-pure structured water and 99.99% pure medical grade silver nanoparticles only, making it much safer than the older forms of silver previously discussed. Quality Assurance is a critical aspect of production and products should be produced in a Certified Good Manufacturing Process (cGMP) facility with FDA inspection and pharmaceutical standards and clean rooms. It is important to distinguish products containing silver from one another. While silver products may be purchased at health food stores, farmer's markets or even produced with silver generators at home, it is important to know that while some of the generators produce a safe colloidal silver, others may be producing inferior quality of ionic silver solutions with much larger silver particles than in the newest structured silver solutions.

Structured silver provides maximum performance

Broadly speaking, unsafe silver products appear in two categories:

those that are impure (silver salts, often combined with an assortment of other elements) and those that are highly concentrated.

By the 2020s, no one should promote the use of impure silver compounds. However, it is a common misperception that many people today insist that more concentrated silver solutions must work better. Yet, researchers at the Brigham Young University Department of Microbiology and Molecular Biology conducted research in 2014 comparing five silver solutions with varying concentrations on their ability to kill a drug-resistant form of Staphylococcus (Methicillin Resistant Staphylococcus Aureus). This study demonstrated that only one of the lower concentration silvers kept pace with a silver that was over 6 times more concentrated.

The demonstrated kill rate of MRSA after 2 minutes:
1. 200 ppm silver- 99.9%
2. 30 ppm structured silver- 99.8%
3. 30 ppm silver- 58.3%
4. 10 ppm silver- 47.1%
5. 10 ppm silver- 39.7%

Two solutions killed nearly all of the bacteria within two minutes while three solutions killed approximately half of the bacteria. Structured silver killed at the maximum rate (over 99%) while older silver technologies (solutions 3, 4, and 5) performed at much lower effectiveness, or relied on an extremely high concentrations (Solution 1) to match the new technology of the structured silver product.

The identity of the non-structured silvers in this study are the decade or century-old technologies mentioned earlier: silver sols, non-structured colloidal silvers and ionic solutions. These remain widely available from many retailers despite their technical inferiority when compared to the newest technology found in the pH balanced, structured silver solutions.

Silver and the body
Silver passes from the body unmetabolized

Not many substances pass through the body unmetabolized, or unchanged from when being swallowed until excreted, but high-quality silver is almost completely eliminated and virtually unmetabolized within 24-48 hours. This is an unusual characteristic of an anti-microbial agent. Pharmaceutical products that work by chemical action are typically consumed by killing germs within the body one molecule at a time until the dose is fully utilized. In contrast, structured silver's ability to work by physics without chemical consumption is a distinguishing characteristic.

The result is that structured silvers are effective at disinfecting on entering the body as it is swished and swallowed, killing the germs associated with gum disease, bad breath and cold sores. Between drinking and excretion, structured silver will be equally effective while travelling through the digestive tract, killing pathogens like E. coli or salmonella that a person may have inadvertently ingested at lunchtime, and also as it is absorbed from the gut, circulating through the bloodstream, killing pathogens in the blood, and even when it is leaving the body, killing the germs that cause bladder and urinary tract infections.

With over 10 million bottles of newer silver solutions consumed in the last decade, no confirmed adverse reaction has been identified. Additionally, immeasurable amounts of colloidal solutions have been safely consumed over the last one hundred years. This is largely connected to the fact that silver, in the right form (pure, metallic and low concentration), passes throughout the body unmetabolized.

Silver and antibiotics

Many people may ask if silver solutions in combination with antibiotics present a problem. Actually, studies have shown that silver solutions have the ability to enhance antibiotic activity greatly when used in combination with antibiotics. Thus, there is no contraindication to the simultaneous use of high-quality silver with antibiotics, only further benefits.

Studies have shown that combining silver with antibiotics resulted in an increased effectiveness of the antibiotics up to 1000 times. Researchers from Harvard theorize that silver disrupts multiple bacterial cellular processes which leads to increased production of reactive oxygen species and increased membrane permeability of even tough, drug-resistant Gram-negative bacteria. This action may potentiate the activity of a broad range of antibiotics against Gram-negative bacteria in different metabolic states, as well as restore antibiotic susceptibility to a resistant bacterial strain.

Key Takeaway: Silver Safety

- High-quality silver is remarkably safe.
- Structured silver solutions selectively kill pathogenic bacteria while leaving the healthy bacteria (probiotics) unharmed.
- Silver is not considered to be a heavy metal.
- Silver is ingested in many foods and found in many body tissues.
- Unsafe silver products appear in two categories: those that are impure and those that are highly concentrated.
- Silver passes from the body unmetabolized.
- Silver is effective from intake through excretion.
- Silver is able to enhance antibiotic activity.

Chapter 4

Silver for Women's Health

Many women will experience gynecologic infections or inflammation, and silver liquid is ideal to use as a cleanse. In the gel form, silver may be used as a topical antimicrobial. Often these infections have become increasingly resistant to antibiotics and antifungal drugs, therefore conventional standard treatments may no longer work for an issue that was once easily treated.

Aging may lead to vaginal dryness, often accompanied by thinning of vaginal tissue. This further may lead to tissue tears which may increase the risk of UTIs and bladder and vaginal infections. Two thirds of women over the age of 60 list vaginal dryness as one of the top five sexual health problems, and it is estimated that 50% of women will experience a bladder infection at least once in their lifetime.

Women's anatomy precludes them to vaginal issues as an increase in gastrointestinal yeast and other microorganisms is associated with increases in contamination due the anatomical proximity of the anus and vulvo-vaginal areas.

Vaginal infections and vaginitis (inflammation) can present either as a yeast infection from an overgrowth of the candida fungus or as a bacterial or viral infection. The symptoms may appear similar, which may lead to a misdiagnosis for treatment.

A Center for Disease Control and Prevention report has shown the number of people infected by chlamydia, gonorrhea, and syphilis is rising. This makes the need for improved feminine hygiene more evident than ever.

Unfortunately, antibiotics prescribed for bacterial infections may in turn cause a vaginal yeast infection, while antifungal drugs for yeast infections may in turn cause a bacterial infection. This unbalanced vaginal microbiome often leaves women fighting a vicious cycle of fungal and bacterial infections.

Research has demonstrated structured silver's antibacterial and antifungal properties. Nanoparticle silver has even been shown to have high therapeutic affect against MRSA, as well as enhancing the antibacterial activity of various antibiotics.

Research has shown the effects of silver inhibiting the replication of Herpes Simplex Virus-2 (HSV-2), concluding that nanoparticle silver solution is a promising treatment for use against sexually transmitted diseases. One study on HIV and HSV-transmitted infections showed that a silver coated polyurethane condom (PUC) may directly inactivate the virus' infectious potential and thus provide another defense against these sexually transmitted microbial infections. The proven success of the antiviral properties of silver on STDs leads to the promising hope for future studies of silver even on Human Papilloma Virus (HPV).

While silver can offer much for all, men and women, the newer pH balanced, structured silvers can *really* make a difference for women's unique health needs.

How can silver help women?

Seven everyday conditions tin which silver may help women include:

1. Bacterial vaginosis: A vaginal infection occurs when more "bad" bacteria are present in the vagina and perineum than "good" bacteria. Silver studies have shown they are able to eradicate the "bad" bacteria while promoting a healthy environment for the "good" bacteria.

2. Vaginal yeast infections: An overgrowth of Candida may infect the vagina, cervix, uterus and vulva. Many symptoms may include foul smell, itching, burning when urinating and abnormal vaginal discharge. Silver solutions have been

shown to destroy yeast in less than 10 minutes and promote and support the "good" microbiome of the vagina.

3. Overall vaginal health: The vagina is a 'self-cleaning' structure, but occasionally it may be overwhelmed. Over washing, using harsh soaps, and not letting the vagina "breathe" from time to time can create an environment that promotes "bad" bacteria and yeast. As silver is antibacterial, antiviral and anti-fungal, the silver liquid and gel are perfect for vaginal cleansing and support.

4. Sexually Transmitted Disease (STD): Exchanging germs during sexual intercourse is inevitable. Unfortunately, your vulva and vagina can be perfect breeding grounds for many microbes passed from your sexual partner. Silver gel is a great sexual lubricant that may be used to increase pleasure and destroy bacteria, viruses or yeast that may be transferred during sexual activity.

5. Urinary Tract Infection (UTI): A urinary tract is bacterial infection that may affect any part of the urinary tract, including the kidneys, ureters, bladder and urethra which may be adversely affected by invading bacteria that multiply in the urine. Taking silver orally and applying silver gel to the vulva may diminish or eliminate the infections.

6. Wounds and inflammation: Wounds may come in many forms and may affect anyone, but it has been noted that women experience higher levels of inflammation than men, which may lead to many chronic disorders. However, a recent study conducted of gene expression showed that silver decreases the expression of many inflammatory genes, while increasing the expression of genes that are associated with wound healing.

7. Gut healing: Functional gastrointestinal (GI) disorders are much more common in women than in men due to fluctuations of female sex hormones. GI disorders include Chron's Disease, Irritable Bowel Syndrome, Gastric Dyspepsia, Proliferated Gastrointestinal Lining Syndrome, Gastric Ulcers and more. Silver solutions may help alleviate

inflammation while supporting the healing of damaged GI tissues. Silver may also eradicate bacterial or fungal pathogens that may be contributing to the gastrointestinal pathologies.

How to use silver for women's health

Some simple ways to use silver for vaginal health:
- Silver may be easily used as a cleansing douche. Pump 2 ounces of silver intravaginally, hold in the vagina for 10-12 minutes and then release. Silver gel may then be applied to the vagina and vulva.
- To receive antibacterial, anti-viral, anti-fungal and even anti-parasitic benefits, apply 2-3 pumps of the gel on a tampon before inserting. This method can be used for 30 minutes at a time, or overnight for HPV positive testing, with appropriate gynecological follow-up evaluations. Preliminary studies are very positive for silver effects to eliminate HPV. Vaginal gel is useful as a sexual lubricant and to enhance general vaginal health.
- In addition to keeping bacterial and yeast infections under control, silver gel may offer protection against bacteria, viruses and other Sexually Transmitted Diseases.
- Silver may be used in the bathtub. Pour 4 ounces silver into a warm bath and soak for 25-30 minutes to help cleanse the vagina, perineum and anus.
- Always take structured silver orally as directed in addition to vaginal use.

Key Takeaway: Silver for Women's Health

- Silver may assist with these 7 everyday issues: bacterial vaginosis, yeast infection, overall vaginal health, Sexually Transmitted Diseases, Urinary Tract Infections, wounds and inflammation and gut healing.
- There are many ways women can incorporate silver into their daily hygiene routine to maintain good health.

Chapter 5

Silver for Animal's Health

While the focus of this writing has been to inform of the many uses of silver for maintaining or regaining health in people, silver may greatly help pets and other animals to enjoy better health as well.

As with people, silver offers a natural therapy for a wide variety of infections and illnesses caused by pathogenic bacteria, viruses, fungi and parasites. A 2016 study conducted at the University of Michigan found that when oral doses of silver nanoparticles were administered for 28 days, the structure and diversity of the animal gut microbiome was maintained. This is in contrast to the detrimental effects of broad-spectrum antibiotics which often eradicate many "good" bacteria (probiotics) in addition to the pathogenic bacteria they are intended to treat.

Why should I use silver with my animals?

Five simple reasons you should use silver with your pets:
1. Silver protects against pathogens: Silver has been shown to effectively eradicate numerous bacteria, viruses, fungi and parasites, many of which are found in pets and other animals.
2. Silver supports the immune system: Silver helps strengthen the immune system against illness and disease.
3. Silver calms digestive ailments: Silver may safely be consumed to help with digestive tract issues such as food poisoning, vomiting, diarrhea and intestinal infections.
4. Silver disinfects pet surroundings: Silver is terrific for disinfecting and cleaning your pets' surroundings, including dog and cat houses, litter boxes, food and water bowls, pet toys, birdcages and more.
5. High-quality pH-balanced, structured silvers are extremely safe. A plethora of studies, as well as thousands of anecdotal cases, have shown silver to be non-toxic and very safe for

internal and external applications in people and animals alike.

How do I use silver with animals?

Silver liquid and gel may destroy the bacteria, viruses, yeast and numerous parasites if the silver solution or gel can stay in contact with the pathogen for six minutes or more. Silver liquid is used for internal consumption (in water bowls, for example), whereas the silver gel is primarily used for external applications because it will stay in place longer. Silver liquid or gel may be added to drinking water, injected into the mouth using a syringe, applied to any surface structure or orifice, and is absorbed very well rectally.

Animals can drink the liquid silver for immune system benefits. Following are amounts proportionate to the body weight of the animal.

For example, a *general oral guideline* may be:
>   <15 pounds: give ½ teaspoon (2.5 ml) twice daily.
>   15-30 pounds: give 1 teaspoon (5 ml) twice daily.
>   30-50 pounds: give 1½ teaspoons (7.5 ml) twice daily.
>   50-80 pounds: give 2 teaspoons (10 ml) twice daily.
>   80-120 pounds: give 2½ teaspoons (12.5 ml) twice daily.
>   120+ pounds: give 1 tablespoon (15 ml) twice daily.

For more serious conditions, or for larger animals, the dose may be doubled or more for several days or a week or more, if clinically indicated.

Silver gel may be given topically, orally and/or in every orifice of the body in doses to cover the wound. Generally, apply twice daily, although it is safe to apply four or more times daily, if clinically indicated.

Key Takeaway: Silver for Animal's Health

- Silver is beneficial for pets and other animals, too.
- Silver protects pets against harmful pathogens.
- Silver supports animals' immune systems.
- Silver assists in digestive issues.
- Silver is a great disinfectant.
- Silver is extremely safe for animals.
- Silver may be administered in water bowls, orally, rectally and directly to wounds.

Chapter 6

Silver & Gut Microbiome Regeneration

"All Disease Begins in the Gut"-Hippocrates

Years of clinical experience with thousands of patients have demonstrated high-quality silver solutions as simply the safest, most efficient and most broad spectrum antimicrobial available.

More recently, functional medicine specialists have again regarded the gastrointestinal tract (GI) as a critical aspect of immunity and health. Silver, too, has been recognized for its impact on GI health.

Since Hippocrates' time nearly 2500 years ago, gut regeneration has now become a top researched topic in health worldwide. With any chronic and/or autoimmune disease, healing the gut is paramount to moving toward health. Everything that is ingested travels from the mouth to the anus through the gut. Curiously, the gut is open at both ends and so the contents never directly come into contact with the internal body. However, the gut impact on the trillions of cells in our bodies is unmistakable.

Through digestion and assimilation of ingested products, our trillions of cells receive nutrition in the form of amino acids, essential fatty acids, minerals and vitamins. Further, the metabolic waste products will be eliminated through the gut, as well as the kidneys and liver.

The GI microbiome (the microbial contents of the gut) is being recognized as a critical factor to maintain or regain health generally. Simply put, trillions of microbes reside in the gut and, in fact, are essential to health and wellbeing. As evidence of the escalating medical research on the gut microbiome, Pub Med showed 74 research articles on the microbiome in 2000 and 9600 in 2017.

Current understanding is that 80%+ of our immune system is located in the gut microbiome. Ninety-five percent of serotonin, the "happy hormone", is produced in the gut along with many other hormones. The GI microbiome digests the ingested foods to produce anti-inflammatory short chain fatty acids, B vitamins and further controls glucose and fat metabolism.

The GI microbiome has far more genes than the rest of the body's own organ and tissue genes. These trillions of gut microbes weigh approximately 3 pounds, similar to our brains. A healthy gut microbiome has approximately 80% "good" microbes (probiotics) and 20% "bad" microbes. When the ratio is skewed with an increase in unhealthy micorbes, the term is "dysbiosis". Small Intestine Bacterial Overgrowth (SIBO) occurs when massive numbers of large intestine microbes invade the small intestine.

Structured silver may be an ideal consideration for both dysbiosis and SIBO as it preferentially destroys pathogenic bacteria and pathogenic yeasts, such as Candida, and stops the replication of both RNA and DNA viruses. However, of great importance, silver, unlike all other pharmaceutical antibiotics, does not damage the lipid cell walls of the good bacteria whereas pathogenic bacteria, which have water soluble cell walls, are thus killed preferentially by the structured silver solution. Studies have further demonstrated benefits for ulcerative colitis as effectively as sulfasalazine, likely due to silver's anti-inflammatory properties.

Silver, along with high quality pro-biotics and pre-biotics, are a great combination for any program to begin to restore gut health.

Key Takeaway: Silver and Gut Regeneration

- The healthy gut supplies the 2 key needs of a healthy cell: Cellular nutrition and cellular excretion.
- Gut health is critical to start and continue whole body healing, including the brain.
- Silver's anti-inflammatory, antimicrobial and immune regulating benefits heal the gut and "leaky gut syndrome" and in turn may initiate whole body healing.
- The microbiome dysbiosis correction, which is absolutely required for health, begins to immediately improve with silver.
- Much supportive material is available to maximize the results silver provides (quality unprocessed food, detox, water, supplements, keto-fasting, exercise, breathing therapy and so on).

Chapter 7

Silver and the Human Genome

Silver has recently been studied on the 20,000+ human genome using ex-vivo human cells. Specifically, pH Structured Silver was studied using a wound healing model to investigate its gene expression effect. The results are a remarkable scientific breakthrough!

Of the 88 genes widely recognized in wound healing, 59 of these genes were regulated with more than a 2-fold expression by the pH Structured Silver solution. Results showed that the pH Structured Silver has amazing anti-inflammatory characteristics as well as gene expressions on the immune system for health benefits.

This research is presently being presented for peer reviewed publication. This is the first silver study of the gene expression on the whole human genome. The results are so profound that silver epigenetic research will likely now expand rapidly worldwide. As just one example, dermcidin (an anti-microbial protein produced in the skin) was expressed over 9-fold by the pH Structured Silver solution. This protein is lacking in the skin of patients with acne and other inflammatory and infectious skin conditions according to published scientific papers. This discovery may lead to critical therapeutic options for patients with the dermcidin deficit.

Another mechanism of action of pH Structured Silver solution may explain why it is so effective against a variety of skin conditions. This includes the anti-inflammatory as well as the antimicrobial and immune regulating characteristics of the silver in the gut. The gut lining is essentially an embryonic skin.

We may assume this breakthrough research of gene expression in wound healing may be extrapolated from superficial skin issues to healing the "leaky gut syndrome", that is healing the outside skin and the inside "skin".

Key Takeaway: pH Structured Silver and the Human Genome

- pH Structured Silver is the only scientifically proven gene expression silver.
- pH Structured Silver applied to wounds produced significant gene expression which in turn enhances the immune and healing responses.
- pH Structured Silver applied to wounds appears to accelerate skin healing.
- Further studies will examine gene expression and therapeutic effects of pH Structured Silver on other "skin" types, such as the vaginal vault and its microbiome as well as the lining and microbiome of the gastrointestinal system.

Chapter 8

Silver for International Travel, Missions and Humanitarian Projects

From: Frank BL. Silver as a Preferred Tool in International Missions and Travel Medicine. In *The Most Precious Metal: Why Silver is More Valuable than Gold, Platinum, or Money. 2nd Edition.* Pedersen G, Ed. Salt Lake City, UT, Silver Health Institute, 2016. (Some editing made by author to update information.)

Introduction

Silver hydrosols of the last decade, and now the even more effective pH balanced, structured silvers, have presented as remarkable therapeutics in many diverse clinical situations in both basic research and clinical experience. Silver demonstrates profound antimicrobial (antibacterial, antiviral, anti-parasitic and antifungal) effects for virtually every surface and tissue of the body. Silver is both highly effective clinically and is non-toxic. These properties make high-quality silver solutions a preferred therapeutic for treating patients, healthcare volunteers and team members in international missions and humanitarian efforts.

International mission efforts often serve those with little or no access to conventional healthcare. Indigenous tribal or traditional remedies are often practiced, some of which are very beneficial. Silver and various silver solutions have been used since antiquity to promote or restore health.

Silver therapies were mentioned in the classic writings of Egyptian health practices over 5500 years ago. Silver was also used by Greeks, Romans, Phoenicians and Macedonians 2500 years ago, with silver vessels for water purification.

Europeans also used silver in order to blunt the effects of the plague through the use of silverware, silver plates and pitchers. In the last two centuries in American medical history, silver has been used in silver sutures, stents and catheters to decrease surgical and procedural infection rates.

Silver kills over 650 different disease-causing organisms! Silver products are now widely used in health care and industry with numerous applications to promote health and wellness. Space stations have used silver-based systems for water purification, as do several commercial airlines. Hospital and hotel environmental systems use silver-based systems to control infections, such as the infamous Legionnaires' Disease. Silver has been used topically for decades in hospitals and clinics for burn victims, diabetic wounds and decubitus ulcers, and is also incorporated into the fabrication of stents that are used in the heart and blood vessels and in the kidneys and urinary tract to decrease infection. Silver is being integrated on various clothing items to decrease body odor or contamination in shirt armpit, caps and socks.

Silver has been shown to interrupt microbes' cell wall function, cellular reproduction, bio-film integrity and other anti-biocide effects.

Additional uses of silver include disinfecting fruits and vegetables and preserving cosmetics, toiletries and similar hygiene products. More US patents have been applied for silver than all other metals combined in recent years, both for health care and for industrial applications. Silver is blended with plastics for lasting anti-microbial protection and in prescription eyeglasses. Silver ions have been demonstrated to promote bone growth in fractures.

Silver-based antimicrobial biocides are used as wood preservatives and to inhibit bacterial growth in chicken farms and oyster harvesting.

With the advanced pH balanced, structured silvers, patients may realize profound benefits and avoid the potential hazards of older and inferior colloidal, ionic and silver salt preparations.

Some traditional cultures (especially in South Asia) have used silver foil as a dietary product for supporting gut health, yct some of the foil is of poor quality and it is not uncommon to see those with argyria (darkening of the skin in a blue-grey coloration) in those using inferior silver products.

Colloidal silver solutions are widely known by many who shop at health food stores, and this was a significant improvement over previous ionic solutions and salts of silver from previous generations. In the last decade or so, silver hydrosols presented even further advancement with smaller silver nanoparticles in suspension, leading to greater penetration on a cellular level.

This chapter is intended to inform of the benefits that may be realized in using structured silver solutions in international travel and humanitarian mission projects. We have found structured silver to be highly effective, non-toxic and therefor extremely safe, and at a good value when compared to expensive pharmaceuticals that are commonly used during international travel.

An integrative missionary and travel physician

This author is a medical missionary with over forty years of experience in a US-based private practice of Anesthesiology, Integrative Pain Management, Anti-aging & Regenerative Medicine, Medical Acupuncture and Advanced Biomagnetics & Bioenergetics, as well as extensive travel medicine and medical missions. In his private medical practice, Dr. Frank is President of *Re-Genesis Health: New Beginnings in Health & Wellness* in Edmond, OK, providing integrative care for pain, metabolic, autoimmune illnesses and more.

As President of *Global Mission Partners, Inc.* (GMP), a 501-c-3 Not-for Profit charitable corporation serving the poor in developing parts of Asia, Africa, South and North America, he has used structured silver for maintaining health and/or treating wide variety of medical condition around the world. He has traveled for missions, teaching or touring to more than 65 countries on 6 continents and his teams currently serve Nepal, Kenya and Mexico. He has also previously served in Russia, Haiti, Ecuador, India, the Dominican Republic, Costa Rica, Appalachia and on Native American reservations.

Dr. Frank has extensive travel and trekking experience, treating team members while on treks in the Himalaya, the Mt. Blanc circuit in Europe or Machu Picchu in Peru, as well as the bustling cities or tiny oxcart villages of Asia, Africa and Latin America. He has authored the Pain Management in Wilderness and Travel Medicine chapter in the renowned and definitive text, Wilderness Medicine, 4th and 5th Editions, and co-authored the 7th Edition Ethnobotany chapter of the same text, edited by the highly acclaimed Stanford Emergency Physician, Dr. Paul Auerbach. He recently co-authored the Prolotherapy chapter in *Neural Therapy Handbook: Therapy with Local Anesthetics* by Georg Thieme Verlag KG publishers of Berlin, 2020. (In German)

As President of Acupuncture Medical Arts, LLC, Dr. Frank has written numerous articles on Medical Acupuncture, Auricular Therapy, Prolotherapy, Neural Therapy, and other related techniques and has published references charts, the Atlas of Auricular Therapy and Auricular Medicine and the acclaimed text, Auricular Medicine and Auricular Therapy: A Practical Approach.
(See www.AuricularTherapy.com)

Dr. Frank has led medical delegations to Russia, China, and Japan for exchanging research and clinical expertise in medical acupuncture. He has lectured across North America and internationally to medical Congresses, Symposia and seminars to many thousands of physicians and other healthcare workers in Europe, Asia, Oceana and North and South America. He served as President of the American Academy of Medical Acupuncture (AAMA) (1999-2001), as President of the International Council of Medical Acupuncture and Related Techniques (ICMART) (2004-2006) and also as Vice-President of ICMART (2002-2004 and 2010-2012).

Dr. Frank is an ordained and licensed pastor and missionary. Over the last 35 years, he has led hundreds of volunteers to serve thousands of needy in over 100 missions for healthcare, care of street children and orphanages, home, clinic and church construction, water-wells, community development, women's skills development, education, micro-loan financing, as well as preaching, teaching and Christian discipleship.

The role of silver in international travel and missions medicine

One role of silver that may be neglected as teams organize and prepare for mission projects is that of preventing disease and maintaining good health in the participants prior to, throughout and following the mission project. With this consideration, the author encourages all adult team members to take 1-2 tablespoons of advanced pH balanced, structured silver solution twice daily in the week prior to the project, continuing throughout and then following, the project for at least one to two weeks (half this dose in children under 12 years age). The continued use after travel is important, as some organisms may be latent and not expressing clinical illness until some days after return from travel.

Silver has great applications for treating patients on the mission field as well. GMP has experience using silver solutions on malaria and typhoid fever in Kenya, upper and lower respiratory infections in Ecuador, skin lesions in India and is used regularly at a Leprosy Mission Hospital in Nepal. The widely effective use of silver for infections from bacteria, viruses, parasites and fungi are seen to be often effective on any surface and any tissue. We have used silver solutions orally, topically as liquid or gel on skin, vagina or rectum, inhaled or sprayed into the nose or mouth and dropped in the eyes and ears. Silver is well received and is without taste and without pain or irritation to body surface or tissues.

It is not uncommon, especially in health camps in primitive "oxcart villages", to be without sophisticated bio-diagnostic tools and instruments. As such, at times a definitive diagnosis is difficult, and

a clinical diagnosis or differential is only available. As silver has a broad spectrum of clinical efficacy, we feel confident in using it when we are unable to finalize a diagnosis. A further benefit is the relative lower cost of high-quality silver solutions compared to many conventional pharmaceuticals.

Many studies show structured silver hydrosols to be safe and effective, and to even enhance antibiotic efficacy against various micro-organisms. Further, with the absence of toxicity, no side effects are to be expected in using advanced silver solutions. This is remarkable, especially when considering the wide range of side effects experienced with many pharmaceuticals, some of which are mild, but there quite serious, even lethal. Hippocrates' charge to, "first, do no harm", may be allowed with ease with high-quality silver solutions, and give comfort to the physician caring for those with little resources to manage serious side effects.

Silver has changed Global Mission Partners' practice of disease prevention for staff and team members over the last decade. In the past, anti-malaria medications or vaccines for yellow fever, typhoid, hepatitis and others would have typically been used. As we now always travel with silver, we do not take the other vaccines and medications as preventatives. It is imperative to take all appropriate precautions to prevent contracting infectious diseases, including but not limited to, thorough hand washing, covering of nose and mouth with coughs and sneezes, thorough washing of utensils and dishes, use of mosquito netting and repellents (natural, non-toxic), where indicated, et cetera.

A challenge to international travel, mission and humanitarian projects

Given the volumes of science, many years of safe experiences with silver, governmental recognitions, the brand spectrum of indications for its use and the reasonable cost value, we strongly encourage international travel and mission agencies and humanitarian projects to seriously consider using a high-quality pH balanced, structured silver on a regular basis for not only the use in field settings or village health camps, but also for staff and personnel in their international placements with regular, daily use of silver for preventive measures, and the daily small use may be increased from 1-2 teaspoons twice daily to 1-2 tablespoons twice daily or more, as indicated, for exposure or onset of illness. In addition, the use of silver gel, drops or sprays may be indicated, depending on the site and clinical presentation of infection.

Silver is not only useful in medical mission projects. Any international travel team or project should seriously consider the benefits of regular, daily silver use as a preventative health measure as well as prompt dosing increase if and when an indicated health problem arises. Simply stated, structured silver is safe, effective and cost-conscious. Management of all companies having personal or other stakeholders' persons in areas known to have infectious disease should make this silver available. It is both morally correct and financially wise.

Stories from the mission fields
Kenya

In a tiny village near of the shores of Lake Victoria, GMP teams have served in health camps, built water wells and latrines, provided meals for orphans and widows with AIDS, and provided education and school support. As we arrived each of the last 15+ years for mission, numerous children and adults in the village presents with illnesses consistent with malaria and/or Typhoid Fever, as well as other co-infections. Malaria is endemic to the region and while diagnosis of the plasmodium parasite in the blood and medications are available, many go without diagnosis and treatment due to extreme poverty. In this setting, GMP uses silver to treat these patients and we hire lab technicians to properly diagnose malaria and Typhoid Fever. Diagnosis is made and patients are then treated with 1-2 tablespoon (15-30 mL) of silver, twice daily. Patients are encouraged to swish the liquid in their mouths for a minute prior to swallowing for absorption to begin across the oral mucous membranes rapidly.

Most patients have been clinically responsive and return to work or school within 24 to 48 hours and their bloodwork for plasmodium or Salmonella typhi have reverted to negative within 2 to 5 days.

Ecuador

Deep in the jungles of southeastern Ecuador, known as el Oriente, is a land that is home to the Shuar indigenous tribal peoples. While Ecuador as roughly 10% of its population from European extraction, approximately 90% are indigenous peoples of approximately 27 different tribes across the nation. Some of these are high mountain peoples, such as the Quichua of the Andes, while others are Amazonian. Unfortunately, the economic reality is inverted, as roughly 90% of the wealth of the nation is in the hands of the minority and only 10% of the wealth is in the hands of the majority of indigenous peoples. Such a situation leads to dire poverty, subsistence living and farming, and lack of basic needs, including medical needs.

The Shuar peoples of el Oriente were head-hunters until a generation or two ago. Now, many live on government protected reservations, much as is seen with many Native American tribal peoples. Yet, without casino gaming, oil and gas and other economic resources as are now going to American Native peoples, this is not the case in Ecuador.

GMP has served in Ecuador for 15 years, first high in the Andes at elevations of 9,000 to 12,000 feet, home of the beautiful Quichua peoples. For three years, GMP has served the Shuar in the cool, dry and gorgeous jungles. In one project, a small boy came to the clinic with a laceration to the foot. While this may be a simple problem for many in North America, lack of health education, even including basic washing and ascpsis, is often unknown in village settings. His infection demonstrated a serious wound was made and silver gel was applied. This was to be reapplied 2-3 times per day, in addition to one tablespoon of liquid structured silver twice daily. The boy experienced clearing of the wound much more rapidly than expected, even from the best of conventional antibiotic care.

In general, applications of silver in Ecuador have included topical wound infections, as well as purulent (pus) eyes, ears and nasal infections. The solution is not painful and has been highly effective when used in place of other optic or otic antibiotic solutions, such as ciprofloxacin or gentamycin drops.

Nepal

The mysterious Kathmandu sits on a high plane, approximately 4,200 feet above sea level, surrounded by a ring of hills at 8,000 to 12,000 feet elevation. On a clear day, free from the usual pollution, the Himalaya show their snowy splendor, reaching 18,000 to 29,035 feet, the southern slopes of Mt. Everest, or Sagarmatha to the Nepali, "Mother Goddess of the Universe".

GMP has served in over 35 missions to Nepal in the last 23 years. On one project, a small girl presented with matting and purulent (pus) drainage from her eyes. These eye infections are highly contagious even in the USA and can spread to all in a family living in a small village homes rapidly as well as to classmates in schools.

Using a small plastic dropper, an advanced pH balanced, structured silver was dropped into both eyes, 2-3 drops each, 2-3 times per day. As with external ear infections, we have seen the silver drops remedy these infections, typically within 24 hours. Further, the drops do not often sting the eye or the ears and thus they are well tolerated.

We have also had patients who do well clinically in Nepal with silver for vaginal and urinary complaints, using the solution both orally and topically, (topical gel for vaginal inflammation or infections). Additionally, our team reports recent successes with Structured Silver gel for psoriasis that was resistant to congenital care.

Beyond these common conditions, we have used silver gel with leprosy patients at a Leprosy Mission Hospital for their very serious wounds which develop due to sensory and motor nerve deficits which accompany this horrible disease. Silver used topically as well as gel or as the solution soaking a gauze on the lesions, as well as oral silver, has demonstrated tissue wound healing that often is better than that seen with conventional pharmaceutical antibiotics and skin wound care products.

Conclusions

Silver solution and gel have proven to be very valuable therapeutics for both the mission health camps and for the health of the team as it travels. Silver's wide range of antibacterial, antiviral, anti-parasitic, anti-fungal and anti-inflammatory properties make it useful for treating many clinical infections. As it is non-painful and can be used orally as well as on anybody surface or in any body opening, there is a wide acceptance for use by patients.

Organizational leaders and travel coordinators should seriously consider the use of an advanced pH balanced, structured silver as the first line of defense for their teams and for their patients. In our situation, we avoid the use of various immunizations and antibiotics and thus their potential side effects due to the success of silver in treating the various infections conditions. Included in this is its use for malaria, where recently anti-malarial medications have demonstrated PTSD-type neurological symptoms.

While we cannot advise anyone to avoid immunizations or antibiotics, and each person should seek the advice of a knowledgeable health care provider, our experience has led us to be confident in this practice whereby we use silver solutions in place of most immunizations and antibiotics. At times, if the silver has not satisfactorily resolved a clinical problem quickly, it may be used in conjunction with other pharmaceuticals with no conflict or harm, in fact, enhancing antibiotic's therapeutic effectiveness. As this is an emerging technology that is not widely known, we encourage all organizational leaders to share the information about silver and its many uses so that their volunteers may be fully informed as to options for their own health as well as that of those they will treat on mission projects.

Please visit www.GlobalMissionPartners.org for further information about Global Mission Partners' efforts around the globe.

Chapter 9

Clinical Applications

From theories to applications

While background information about silver may be interesting, the real excitement occurs when we first experience silver working in our own lives. While detail for specific situations is helpful, it is also helpful to start with a general recommendation for silver use. In most cases, a good plan is to drink 1-2 tablespoons (15-30 ml) of liquid silver twice daily and to apply gel or liquid topically as needed. There are more specific recommendations that can be more helpful, but generally speaking a good rule of thumb is: "two tablespoons, twice daily; gel as needed."

For severe, life-threatening infections, doctors have recommended as much as 2 ounces every six hours until there is evidence that the infection has been overcome. Silver is also synergistic with antibiotics; thus, it increases the efficiency of prescribed antibiotics and is not in competition with them. Silver and antibiotics are safe to take together!

Many people like to use gel for topical applications, but the liquid can be applied topically as well. Pocket-sized spray containers, cotton balls, gauze and soaking are all easy ways to gain topical benefit of silver using the liquid, if the gel is unavailable.

Before diving into more specific applications, remember to have open conversations with your physician about silver use. If they are unfamiliar with the benefits of silver, ask them to research the enormous volume of research available on the internet on silver's antimicrobial effects for more information. Great physicians never stop learning and should not be threatened by information that may benefit their patients even when it is "alternative" to their conventional understanding.

One product, many pathogens, many locations

Structured silver has hundreds of uses and provides a quantum leap in the treatment and prevention of many health problems. Whether it is used for life-threatening infections such as a drug-resistant superbug pneumonia or sepsis, for protection from epidemics, or for something as superficial as Athlete's Foot, the list of benefits is long.

In addition, cascading health benefits may also occur in seemingly unrelated ways. For example, silver is an excellent tool for improving the health of the gut microbiome, or the collection of microorganisms within the digestive tract. By improving the microbiome, profound health changes include mental health, autoimmune disease, weight loss and digestion become possible. Read Chapter 6, Silver & Gut Microbiome Regeneration in this book for more insight on healing from the inside outward.

Skeptics and even conscientious readers may be wary of such statements. The following pages explain how one product can have hundreds of uses and why every person you know should have a high-quality structured silver solution in their First Aid Kit for everyday protection or for crisis management.

Silver has a broad spectrum of activity, meaning it kills many types of pathogens. Moreover, each of these pathogens can flourish in a wide range of our anatomy, such as eyes, ears, brain, heart, skin, gastrointestinal tract or genitals. Therefore, silver kills germs that may grow in many different locations.

Some may now ask, "well what about something like boils or conjunctivitis, can silver help with those diseases?" Boils and pustules are infections in the skin and conjunctivitis ("Pink Eye") is an infection in the eye. These may seem like two distinct ailments, but they are both infections caused by the same Staphylococcus aureus pathogenic bacteria. Research has shown that silver can kill Staphylococcus aureus, whether it be on the skin or in the eye.

Now consider an otitis, sinusitis and bronchitis. Each is an infection, otitis of the ear, bronchitis of the bronchial tubes of the lungs, sinusitis of the sinuses (hollow cavities in the skull). Each of these infections (with Greek suffix origins) refer to an inflammation (-*itis*) in a specific location. Further, each of these infections in their differing locations may be infected with the same pathogenic bacteria, Staphylococcus pneumoniae. Research has demonstrated that silver can kill this pathogen, no matter its location. Therefore, silver may help your ear infection, your sinus infection and your bronchitis. Further, different diseases of the same location may be associated with different pathogens. For example, bronchitis and pneumonia may be caused by an overgrowth of Staphylococcus aureus, Haemophilus influenzae, Pseudomonas aeruginosa, Streptococcus pneumoniae and others.

As the above infectious diseases are mentioned where silver may be as or more effective than conventional antibiotics or used in addition to the antibiotics, always seek qualified healthcare professionals for serious and life-threatening infections.

General considerations

This section provides more detailed information for using silver solutions with various infectious ailments that we may encounter daily. This list of applications is not comprehensive but is a good guideline for everyday situations.

These statements have not been evaluated by the FDA, nor is this book or this product intended to cure, treat, diagnose, or prevent any disease. Every person's health situation is unique, and no book can substitute for medical care. The best action for your health is using this book to have an open conversation with your doctor or trusted health professional about your personal situation.

Antibacterial

Billions of bacteria are found on the skin, in the bloodstream, the intestines, the hair, and these may be pathogenic or disease-causing bacteria. When examined in the laboratory, studies show that serious chronic diseases are associated with the presence of a pleiomorphic (changes form) bacteria or mold. These pathogenic microbes damage the immune function that normally protects the cells from foreign invaders. When the bacteria or mold invade a cell and reduce this protection, they allow toxins to enter the cell and damage the DNA, allowing serious disease to initiate. Silver begins killing bacteria in as little as 15 seconds. Studies reveal that placing silver gel, liquid or mist in direct contact with bacteria will usually destroy the bacteria within six minutes. Some bacteria may take longer but can be destroyed with regular silver use.

For preventive use of bacterial infections, consider drinking 1-2 teaspoons of liquid silver twice daily. This dose may be doubled or more to fight an aggressive bacterial infection. Silver gel maybe apply topically to any affected areas 1 to 4 times a day. Immune supporting herbs and/or homeopathic remedies may also be beneficial for immune support.

Silver gel is currently being used in clinical trials. Results are showing that it can help close deep open-tunneling wounds, leprotic wounds and Staphylococcus infections, including MRSA. By spraying the liquid solution or applying gel on the wound 2-4 times daily, bacteria are destroyed, and the body can heal itself more quickly.

Antiviral

Viruses cause many diseases, and we only have a few pharmaceutical drugs to treat viruses. Often viral infections are treated incorrectly with antibiotics, which are indicated for bacterial infections but do nothing to destroy or cure viral infections. Silver acts very powerfully against both DNA and RNA viruses, interfering with the viral replication process.

A virus is constructed of a capsid which contains segments of DNA and RNA. These DNA segments carry a slight magnetic charge. There is a "claw" on the virus that attaches the virus to a healthy cell. Once the virus is attached to a healthy cell, it can 'inject' the

DNA or RNA segments into the healthy cell, hijacking your cell's natural cell building machinery, causing your cell to make more viruses.

Silver acts like a magnet that attracts the charged DNA or RNA particles. The DNA or RNA binds so tightly to the silver that the cell makes a chaotic tangle of incomplete genetic material that cannot complete the replication process and thus inactivates the virus.

To prevent a cold or flu, drink 1-2 teaspoons of silver twice daily. When exposed to coughing and sneezing, the dose may be doubled. Silver taken 2 tablespoons twice daily will typically help defeat an existing viral infection quite rapidly. Inhaling a nebulized form of silver works best for a viral infection in the lungs, bronchi or sinuses. Drops can also be placed in your eyes, ears, nose or throat 2-4 times daily.

Antifungal

Fungi thrive in warm, moist areas and typically feed on sugars. Significant reductions in dietary sugars and simple carbohydrates are critical to combat intestinal fungus or yeast. For fungal infections in the axillae (armpits) or vagina, apply silver gel directly to the area 2-4 times daily and take liquid silver orally. High quality probiotics supplementation may be used helpful as well to help reestablish a health gut microbiome.

Intestinal fungus and yeast may be associated with muscle pains, fatigue and symptoms of depression and Attention Deficit/Hyperactivity Disorders, as well as headaches, fibromyalgia, lupus and other auto-immune disorders.

Many people have resolved fungal symptoms by taking 1-2 tablespoons of silver twice daily as a part of their intestinal fungus and yeast cleanse. The cleanse may be accompanied by one to three weeks of flu-like symptoms while fungus and yeast and toxins are eliminated. Silver instilled in the rectum and vaginal as douches have aided many with fungus and yeast in those areas.

Antiparasitic

Parasites are organisms which, unlike bacteria and viruses, present with some species that are microscopic while other species visible with the unaided eye. Parasitic infections are widespread around the globe and represent some of the deadliest infections or infestations in mankind.

The World Health Organization estimates that one fourth people have a chronic parasitic infection of some kind. Parasites may be in the intestines, under the skin or in the lungs or other organs. Parasites can come from the food we eat, including pork and fish, especially when undercooked or raw. Once inside the body, the parasites lay eggs, which hatch and take up residence in the body and then the process is repeated.

Common parasitic infections world-wide include Malaria, African Sleeping Sickness, Amebiasis, Anisakis, Ascaris, Babesia, Balantidium, Bed Bugs, Body Lice, Chagas Disease, Guinea Worm Disease, Tapeworm, Filaria, Entamoeba, Fasciola, Filaria, Giardia, Loa loa, Hookworm, Leishmania, Mite (Scabies), Toxoplasma, Trichinella and many others.

Malaria is a mosquito-borne infectious disease that affects humans and other animals. The parasites Plasmodium falciparum, P. vivax, P. ovale, P. malariae, P. knowlesi are transmitted from infected mosquitoes to people and animals. Outbreaks are increased in rainy seasons when standing, stagnant waters lead to heavy breeding of the mosquitoes.

Malaria is one of the greatest killers on the planet. Malaria causes symptoms that typically include fever, fatigue, vomiting and headaches. Serious infections are seen globally, and the World Health Organization estimates that in 2018, 228 million clinical cases of malaria occurred, and 405,000 people died of malaria.

Studies have demonstrated a high success rate in treating malaria with oral silver 1-2 tablespoons twice daily, with eradication of the Plasmodium parasite in the peripheral blood smear within 2-5 days.

Continue the routine for 2 weeks if symptoms persist or relapse.

While studies have not been performed on many of the parasites and the effect of silver solutions, given the seriousness of the parasitic infections and the safety of high-quality structured silver solutions, it seems prudent to consider using silver as it has been demonstrated helpful in the treatment of malaria and for other parasitic infections as well.

Clearly, qualified medical consultation is essential in these potentially serious and life-threatening illnesses.

Anti-inflammatory

The anti-inflammatory effects of structured silver are much less well known. Gene expressions studies for the first time show the reason behind the anti-inflammatory effects of structured silver. Clinically these effects are seen rapidly in eye and ear infections, wound recovery treatment of burns. Inflammation and chronic disease, especially of the GI tract are well understood to be a significant contributor to auto-immune conditions.

Specific applications for everyday use

While it is not practical to address every clinical case that may respond well to silver, the following list may provide a guide for those with the various symptoms below. While many or most of these infections may be addressed with silver alone, or in combination with herbal/botanicals, homeopathic remedies or other immune supporting measures, *all patients with serious or life-threatening infections should seek qualified healthcare consultation along with the use of silver.*

Head and neck
Bad breath/halitosis

Bad breath or halitosis is usually the result of bacteria residing in the mouth, gums, throat or between teeth. A silver rinse and/or gargle may effectively destroy these bacteria. The rinse and/or gargle is best for 1-2 minutes twice daily, swallowing the silver solution afterward.

Canker sores/aphthous ulcers

Canker sores are typically small, shallow round or oval lesions with a white or yellow center and a red border. They generally form inside the cheeks, on or under the tongue, at the base of the gums or on the soft palate at the roof of the mouth. They may cause a tingling or burning sensation a day or two before the sores actually appear.

Canker sores may be triggered by a minor injury in the mouth, overzealous brushing or by an accidental cheek bite. Mouth rinses and/or toothpastes that include sodium lauryl sulfate as well food sensitivities, spicy or acidic foods may also predispose one to canker sores. Vitamin deficiencies, including B-12, zinc, folate or iron and emotional stresses or hormonal shifts during women's cycles may aggravate canker sores. Helicobacter pylori, the same cause of peptic (stomach) ulcers, and less commonly Herpes simplex virus, may lead to canker sores, as well as immune suppression from any cause.

Silver can help improve oral health quickly. The silver rinse and/or gargle is best for 1- 2 minutes twice daily, swallowing the silver solution afterward. Additionally, silver gel may be applied topically to the lesions for added benefit.

If the canker sore is a result of the herpes virus, the sooner you apply the gel to the wound, the sooner you can stop the virus from replicating and getting worse. You may expect the wound to improve twice as fast with silver gel applied to the canker sore than if it were to run its course naturally.

Cold sores/fever blisters

Cold sores are a common viral infection of Herpes simplex virus (Type 1 commonly, Type 2 at times) causing tiny fluid-filled blisters on or around the lips. The sores may be single or in clusters and will form a scab as the blisters break. Without therapy, most cold sores will heal in 2-3 weeks. Some prescription or OTC remedies may diminish the duration of the lesions, yet silver applied promptly on emergence of the sensitivity that often precedes the appearance of actual lesions may, in fact, even prevent the emergence of the lesions.

Take 1-2 tablespoons of silver solution 2-3 times daily during outbreaks and use silver gel to the lesions 2-4 times daily.

Conjunctivitis/Pink Eye

Conjunctivitis is an inflammation of the eye and lid often associated with viral or bacterial infections. Typically, the sclera (the white of the eye) and the inner lids are red and inflamed. Conjunctivitis can be very painful and if not treated rapidly may lead to serious infections.

Silver has demonstrated highly effective and rapid clearing of conjunctivitis for many. Apply two to three drops of silver eye drops liquid directly into the eyes two to four times daily. Silver gel may also be placed directly into the eyes where the gel will stay in place longer. Additionally, drink 1-2 teaspoons (child) or 1-2 tablespoons (adult) twice a day until the problem is resolved.

Dental health and cavities

Cavities in the teeth develop as the hard enamel surface of the tooth is corroded by sugars and bacteria, commonly seen in dental plaque. Regular rinsing the mouth with silver will dramatically diminish the cavity-causing bacteria and retard plaque development. Rinse the mouth with 1-2 teaspoons of silver twice daily then swallow afterward.

Ear infections/otitis

Ear infections are the result of viral and bacterial infections in the middle ear or external ear canal. Otitis may be associated with other illnesses, including the common cold, flu or sore throat/pharyngitis. Overuse of antibiotics has led to drug resistant bacteria for many patients.

Often patients will rapidly clear their ear infections with structured silver solution, 1-2 teaspoons twice daily for a child and with 2-3 drops in each ear 2-4 daily, as well, allowing the drops to stay in the ear canals for several minutes each before changing position. Daily Vitamin D3 and Vitamin C are important to increase resistance to these infections. Additionally, chewing gum or mints with xylitol twice daily has been demonstrated to decrease the frequency of middle ear infections in children.

Sinus congestion/sinusitis

Nasal and sinus congestion can range from bothersome stuffiness to serious infections. Spraying 2-3 puffs of silver intranasally, followed by deep inhalation, may help protect the nose and sinuses from developing a bacterial, viral or fungal infection or clearing those that have developed. Spray each nostril 2-4 times daily and then inhale deeply. In addition, drink 1-2 teaspoon (child) or 1-2 tablespoons (adult) of silver twice daily to reduce sinusitis, cold and nasal congestion. Gargle and swish the silver solution for about a minute then swallow.

Sore throat/pharyngitis

Sore throats or pharyngitis are commonly caused by viruses and less often by bacteria. Cold and flu viruses are common infections that are associated with sore throat and "Strep throat" is commonly related to a Group A Beta Streptococcal infection.

Rinse and gargle 1-2 teaspoons (child) or 1-2 tablespoons (adult) of silver solution for 1-2 minutes twice daily, swallowing the silver solution afterward. Also, use 2-3 sprays of silver nasal spray in each nostril, deeply inhaled, 2-4 times daily.

Tonsillitis

Tonsillitis is the inflammation of the tonsils caused by bacteria and viruses. Recurrent tonsillitis is often treated surgically by removal of the tonsils. This is unfortunate because tonsils are a key organ in the immune system.

Gargle 1-2 teaspoons (child) or 1-2 tablespoons (adult) for 1-2 minutes 2-3 times each day, will help decrease the bacteria and viruses. Spraying silver into the nostrils 2-3 times daily will also help. Often the pain of pharyngitis will rapidly diminish with the silver gargles, many times within 10-15 minutes.

Chest and abdomen
Acid reflux/heart burn

Acid reflux is often referred to as heartburn. It is commonly thought to occur when too much stomach acid pools in the stomach and then refluxes back into the esophagus. Studies show that for most, there is actually *decreased* stomach acid, leading to poor digestion of stomach contents which then lead to irritability and the subsequent reflux action. While the pH (acidity) of the stomach is not sufficient for its digestive purposes in the stomach, the pH is much more acidic than the esophagus tolerates and thus the discomfort that is experienced.

Silver may be taken daily to help acid reflux symptoms. Take 1-2 teaspoons, two to four times daily as needed. The current recommendation in functional medicine may also include taking 1-2 capsules of digestive aids with each meal, containing Betaine HCl, bile and digestive enzymes.

Asthma

Asthma occurs when the small airways in the lungs become inflamed and restrict air flow, decreasing the amount of air going into the lungs. Asthma often presents with wheezing, coughing, choking and mucus production that can lead to anxiety and decreased oxygenation.

Asthma patients often benefit when they inhale silver from a nebulizer for fifteen minutes 2-3 times daily. Additionally, 1-2 teaspoons (child) or 1-2 tablespoons (adult) of silver solution twice daily may greatly benefit asthma patients.

Bronchitis

Bronchitis is a viral or bacterial infection of the bronchi, the small airways in the lungs. Bronchitis typically results and excess mucus production, congested lungs and coughing.

Drink 1-2 teaspoons (child) or 1-2 tablespoons (adult) of silver 2-4 times daily and inhale silver solution from a nebulizer for fifteen minutes twice daily, along with nasal spray 2-4 times daily, followed by deep inhalation of the silver.

Colds/flu

Colds and flu are viral infections. The viruses enter the nose and possibly the sinuses and replicate, often producing a lot of mucus.

Take 1-2 teaspoons (child) or 1-2 tablespoons (adult) of silver solution three times daily and use the silver nasal spray 3-4 times daily to help reduce the congestion and inflammation and viral load. Oral rinses, eardrops, eyedrops, nose drops, and throat spray may all be used as indicated.

Colitis, diverticulitis, Irritable Bowel Syndrome (IBS)

Colitis is inflammation of the large intestine or colon. Irritable Bowel Syndrome is characterized by inflamed bowels, and with alternating constipation and diarrhea. Diverticulitis is a condition where small outpouchings in the colon become inflamed and/or infected. Referral to a qualified medical practitioner is important and silver solution may be used alongside pharmaceutical remedies, if prescribed.

Take 1-2 tablespoons of silver (adult) 2-3 times daily for acute conditions and 1-2 times daily for maintenance.

Food poisoning

Food poisoning typically includes symptoms such as nausea, vomiting, abdominal cramping and diarrhea. It occurs suddenly (within 48 hours) after consuming a contaminated food or drink, usually caused by bacteria and viruses.

To fight food poisoning requires aggressive silver solution use, drinking about one to two ounces immediately, followed by two tablespoons every hour for the next eight hours. For prevention, drink 1-2 teaspoons 2-3 times daily. This can be especially helpful when travelling to a foreign country.

You may spray silver solution on food to kill the pathogens and possibly prevent food poisoning. After spraying on the food, let it stand for several minutes before eating.

Gastritis, gastric ulcers, gas

Gas can be produced from yeast and sugar mixing with fruits and vegetables in your intestines. Intestinal gas can also be produced directly from certain fruits, vegetables and bacteria. Beans and other legumes, such as peas and lentils, have a reputation for causing gas. Beans contain high amounts of a complex sugar called oligosaccharide, which the body has difficulty breaking down.

Oligosaccharides in beans are propelled to the large intestine undigested. Bacteria in the large intestine finally break down these sugars. This bacterial activity causes fermentation and the production of gas that we release as flatulence. Beans are also rich in fiber, which may increase intestinal gas.

Silver taken orally 1-2 tablespoons twice daily may decrease gas production and one may consider 1-2 capsules with each meal of digestive enzymes, Betaine HCl and bile salts, if indicated.

Gastric (stomach) ulcers are caused by a bacterium called Helicobacter pylori (H. pylori), which injures the lining of the stomach, sometimes leading to a bleeding ulcer. Taking 1-2 tablespoons of silver solution 2-3 times daily may greatly improve gastritis or ulcer conditions.

Pelvis
Bladder infection

Bladder infections are more common in women, due to the short urethra from the bladder to the external body. Bacteria around the urethral opening in the perineum may ascend the urethra and lead to a bladder infection quite rapidly. Bladder infections may become serious very quickly and many women will feel quite sick with fever, chills, nausea, achiness and more. Serious bladder infections may ascend the ureters from the bladder to the kidneys, causing kidney infections.

Drink 2 tablespoons of silver hourly for the first two days. As symptoms subside, take 2 tablespoons silver twice daily. Additionally, many women find great relief with d-mannose, a sugar that binds to the bacteria, forming a complex that does not attach to the bladder wall and is thus eliminated with urination. Cranberry juice or capsules often help women's bladder health as well.

Diaper rash

When babies wear diapers, their skin may be in contact with urine or stool for long periods of time. This warm, moist area of the skin will allow bacteria and fungus to grow very quickly. The skin becomes red and may even crack or bleed. Silver gel applied generously to the diaper rash often reduces the problem quite quickly, including the redness and pain.

To help prevent diaper rash, spray a thin layer of silver on the inside of the diaper and allow it stand for several minutes before putting on the baby. Silver gel applied regularly will also help many babies avoid further diaper rash.

Diarrhea/dysentery

Diarrhea may be caused by bacteria, viruses or parasites. Dysentery is an infection of the intestines resulting in severe diarrhea with the presence of blood and mucus in the stools. The cause of dysentery is usually the bacteria Shigella, in which case it is known as shigellosis, or the amoeba, Entamoeba histolytica. Other causes may include certain chemicals, other bacteria, protozoa or parasitic worms.

Take 1-2 teaspoons of silver twice daily to help prevent diarrhea, especially when traveling. If you experience diarrhea or dysentery, take 2 tablespoons of silver solution every hour for the first six to eight hours. As symptoms improve, take the silver solution 3-4 times daily for several days. Probiotics to replenish the healthy bacteria of the gut are also recommended.

Genital infections/Sexually Transmitted Disease (STD)

Sexually Transmitted Diseases (STD) are infections passed from one person to another through sexual contact. You may contract an STD by having unprotected vaginal, anal or oral sex with someone who has the STD. The most common sexually transmitted infections in the United States are HPV, chlamydia and gonorrhea.

Protected sex is of primary importance in preventing spread of STD. Once one has an STD, silver gel applied topically may help the STD outbreak improve more quickly and should be applied 2-4 times daily as soon as the outbreak occurs. In addition, drink 2 teaspoons of silver twice daily to help prevent future outbreaks.

For women who test positive for HPV, some HPV tests have reverted to normal with a nightly insertion of silver gel on a tampon, removed each morning and continued for a month. Additionally, vaginal cream applicators are available for insertion of structured silver application intravaginally. Pump the gel 2-3 times via the applicator twice per day. Finally, silver gel is a recommended personal lubricant useful for sexual activity.

Musculoskeletal
Arthritis

Arthritis is characterized by painful swelling and inflammation of the joints. The most common arthritis is generalized degenerative or osteoarthritis, simply a "wear and tear" process from aging, injuries or accidents.

Gout is a common and complex form of arthritis characterized by sudden, severe attacks of pain, swelling, redness and tenderness in the joints, often the joint at the base of the great toe. Gout is caused by a condition known as hyperuricemia, or excess uric acid in the body. Foods and drinks that often trigger gout attacks include organ meats, game meats, some types of fish, fruit juice, sugary sodas and alcohol. On the other hand, fruits, vegetables, whole grains, soy products and low-fat dairy products may help prevent gout attacks by lowering uric acid levels.

Rheumatoid arthritis is a chronic inflammatory disorder resulting from an autoimmune disorder, caused by the immune system attacking healthy body tissue.

To lessen the pain of arthritis, drink 1-2 teaspoons silver twice daily. Silver gel may also be applied topically to the joint if it is hot or red. Glucosamine, chondroitin sulfate, hyaluronic acid and essential fatty acids may also be helpful.

Skin
Abscesses/cysts

Abscesses and cysts are pockets of bacterial infection in the skin or other tissues. Silver gel may be applied liberally to the abscess and gently rubbed into the tissue for 30-60 seconds 3-4 times daily. Oral silver, 2 tablespoons 2-3 times daily may enhance healing. Many abscesses will clear within just a few days using silver, however, if symptoms worsen or red streaking appears from the abscess, qualified medical practitioners may find a need to incise and drain the abscess. The silver gel and oral intake may be continued even if conventional antibiotic care is required.

Acne

Acne attacks people of all ages, from infants to adults. Bacteria inside a hair follicle or a sweat gland, called a sebaceous gland, can cause acne. Please see in Chapter 7 that pH Structured Silver studies show an increase in dermcidin by 9-fold. Research shows acne patients lack dermcidin in their skin.

Many people see clearing of acne by applying silver gel liberally to the skin 2-3 times daily, (may be applied before makeup) and taking 1-2 tablespoons of silver orally twice daily.

Age spots

Age spots are small, flat dark areas on the skin. They vary in size and usually appear on areas exposed to the sun, such as the face, hands, arms and shoulders. Age spots may also be called sun spots, liver spots and solar lentigines.

Some have reported success in lightening the age spots with taking 1-2 teaspoons of silver twice daily and applying silver gel twice daily.

Athlete's Foot

Athlete's Foot, or tinea pedis, is a fungal infection that usually begins between the toes. It commonly occurs in people whose feet have become sweaty while confined in shoes. Signs and symptoms of athlete's foot include a scaly rash, itching, stinging and burning.

The first step to prevention is to wear clean shoes and socks and reduce the amount of time that your feet stay in a moist sock or shoe.

Silver may be sprayed into your socks and shoes to kill bacteria. Allow to dry for 5 minutes before wearing. Apply silver gel between the toes and/or on the toenails. Finally, soak the feet for 30 minutes daily or every other day in a silver bath to help with difficult cases.

Bites, insects, spiders

Bug, insect and spider bites and stings often introduce both toxins and bacteria. Silver helps by reducing inflammation and pain and improves wound healing.

Apply silver gel immediately and 3 times daily. Drink 2 tablespoons of silver twice daily for 3-4 days as the bite or sting resolves.

Burns/sunburn

Burns may occur from the sun's radiation, x-rays, fire, heat and chemicals in our environment. Silver is often highly effective to help treat a burn. Silver reduces pain and inflammation and improves wound healing. Silver liquid can be sprayed on the burn or used to soak the burn. Silver gel may be applied to the wound 3-4 times daily and will often demonstrate decrease in redness and tenderness or pain quite quickly. Additionally, silver therapies have been applied for many decades in hospitals and clinics for burns, commonly in the form of silver sulfadiazine. Structured silver solution and gel will likely aid these patients very well to both heal more quickly and to prevent infections.

Drink 2 tablespoons of silver liquid twice daily until the burn has subsided and apply silver gel liberally to the skin burn. This may also help prevent infection in the burn.

Chicken pox

Chicken pox, also called Herpes zoster or Varicella zoster, is a common, highly contagious viral infection that causes an itchy rash with small, fluid-filled blisters. Once infected, the virus will reside in the body for the rest of one's life. If the body's natural immune antibody response is compromised, shingles may develop as the virus is reactivated and travels from the posterior spinal cord out along peripheral nerves. Typically, shingles develops as a swath of blisters around the chest or abdomen, less commonly on the face or inguinal regions. These lesions may be very painful and chronic complications of Post-herpetic Neuralgia (post shingles pain) are increased with each decade of life beyond the 60s.

With either Chicken pox or shingles, gently apply the gel liberally to the lesions 3-4 times daily. Drink 2 teaspoons (child) or 2 tablespoons (adult) of silver solution twice daily. For adults who think they are getting shingles, but do not yet see the lesions, the gel may be applied directly to the skin that is painful.

Wounds/ulcers/bed sores

Wounds may include burns, cuts, abrasions, ulcers or bed sores, bruises or broken bones. Silver solutions have been documented to help improve wound healing. In a study done at the University of Utah, pigs healed substantially faster and had less bacteria, viruses and mold when treated with silver.

Gene markers have demonstrated proof of gene expressions of anti-inflammatory action of silver, which may greatly facilitate healing of wounds more quickly. See Chapter 7, Silver and the Human Genome.

Apply silver gel to any wound, open or closed, 3-4 times daily. Keeping the wound moist and covered with either silver solution soaked gauze or silver gel will enhance healing. Drink 1-2 teaspoons to 1-2 tablespoons of silver solution twice daily to help prevent or treat bacterial contamination of wounds.

Systemic Epidemics/pandemics

Epidemic outbreaks, either bacterial, viral or parasitic, are common. These have may include the annual cold and influenza outbreaks, Bird Flu, Zika, Chikungunya, West Nile Virus, Ebola and others.

Take 1-2 teaspoons (child) or 1-2 tablespoons (adult) of advanced structured silver solution twice daily for outbreaks, or even to help prevent illness if not yet infected. Silver liquid or gel is very effective as a hand sanitizer and should be used liberally and often. Silver liquid may also be used to help keep water purified, with 32 ounces in a 55-gallon barrel of water for storage.

Silver liquid may be used topically, nasally, inhaled as nebulized, intravaginally or rectally. Any or all of these methods should be considered in the event of an epidemic, as indicated.

Inflammation/swelling

Inflammation and swelling may be due to trauma or from bacteria, viruses, parasites or fungus. Apply silver liquid or gel liberally to inflammation and swelling 2-3 times daily and drink 1-2 teaspoons (child) or 1-2 tablespoons (adult) silver liquid twice daily.

Lyme Disease

Lyme disease is a bacterial infection from the bite of an infected tick belonging to a few species of the genus Ixodes ("hard ticks"). The disease is caused by the bacterium Borrelia burgdorferi and rarely, Borrelia mayonii. At first, Lyme disease usually causes symptoms such as a rash, fever, headache and fatigue. If not treated early, the infection may lead to symptoms of the joints, heart and nervous system.

Clinical manifestations of Lyme disease are divided into three stages:
1. Flu-like symptoms and a Bull's Eye-type skin rash (Erythema Migrans). Some people, however, develop a different rash or perhaps no rash at all.
2. Weeks or months later, Bell's Palsy or meningitis type neurological symptoms may develop.
3. Months to years later, systemic arthritis may develop.

Symptoms may progressively increase if the disease is not effectively treated.

Physicians usually prescribe antibiotics such as doxycycline, cefuroxime or amoxicillin for Lyme Disease. These may be fairly effective if given early, within the first two weeks of infection, but the efficacy may diminish overtime due to the progressive nature of the disease.

If you know (or think) you have been bitten by a tick within the past two weeks, drink 1-2 teaspoons (child) or 1-2 tablespoons (adult) of silver twice daily and apply silver gel to the bite four times daily for two weeks.

If you have Lyme Disease, drink 4 tablespoons of high-quality structured silver liquid twice daily and apply silver gel to the affected or sore areas twice daily. Continue this for three months, then reduce the dose by half for a month and return to full dose for a month and continue if needed.

Malaria and other parasites

Malaria is a mosquito-borne infectious disease that affects humans and other animals. The parasites Plasmodium falciparum, P. vivax, P. ovale, P. malariae, P. knowlesi are transmitted from infected mosquitoes to people and animals. Outbreaks are increased in rainy seasons when standing, stagnant waters lead to heavy breeding of the mosquitoes.

Malaria is one of the greatest killers on the planet. Malaria causes symptoms that typically include fever, tiredness, vomiting, and headaches. Serious infections are seen globally, and the World Health Organization estimates that in 2018, 228 million clinical cases of malaria occurred, and 405,000 people died of malaria.

Further, recent studies reveal that some of the Post Traumatic Stress Disorder (PTSD) symptoms demonstrated in soldiers who have spent time in the Middle East are actually side effects of the malaria pharmaceutical prophylaxis, such as Lariam (brand name for mefloquine). The use of an effective therapy and preventative solution of silver seems prudent as it is without these serious side effects.

Studies have shown a high success rate in treating malaria with oral silver solution 1-2 tablespoons twice daily, with eradication of the Plasmodium parasite in the peripheral blood smear within 2-5 days. Continue the routine for 2 weeks if symptoms persist or relapse. Importantly, as a community begins to clear malaria infections in the people, there is less malaria load within the community for mosquitos to acquire the parasite and then infect other animals and people. This gradual diminishing or eradication of malaria load leads not only to enhanced health within the communities but also greatly furthers the education of the children and youth as they miss fewer days of schooling due to illness and graduation rates and school marks have progressively accelerated in our communities in Kenya through this approach with silver.

The World Health Organization estimates that one fourth of people have a chronic parasitic infection of some kind. Parasites may be in the intestines, under the skin or in the lungs or other organs. Parasites can come from the food we eat, including pork and fish, especially when undercooked or raw. Once inside the body, the parasites lay eggs, which hatch and take up residence in the body and then the process is repeated.

Common parasitic infections world-wide include African Sleeping Sickness, Amebiasis, Anisakis, Ascaris, Babesia, Balantidium, Bed Bugs, Body Lice, Chagas Disease, Guinea Worm Disease, Tapeworm, Filaria, Entamoeba, Fasciola, Filaria, Giardia, Loa loa,

Hookworm, Leishmania, Mite (Scabies), Toxoplasma, Trichinella and many others.

While studies have not been performed on many of the parasites and the effect of silver solutions, given the seriousness of the parasitic infections and the safety of structured silver, it seems prudent to consider using silver as it has been demonstrated helpful in the treatment of malaria and for other parasitic infections as well.

Clearly, qualified medical consultation is essential in these potentially serious and life-threatening illnesses.

References

General silver references:

Holladay RJ, et al. Treatment of humans with colloidal silver composition. United States Patent No. 7,135,195 B2, Nov 14, 2006.

Silvestry-Rodriguez N, et al. Silver as a Disinfectant. Rev Environ Contam Toxicol 191:23-45.

Khan S, et al. Nanosilver: new ageless and versatile biomedical therapeutic scaffold. *Int J Nanomed* 2018:13:733-762.

Bhayani, R. India's silver use triples in a decade, world share up from 14.7% to 39.2%. *Business Standard.* [Online] June 14, 2018. [Cited: November 15, 2020.] https://www.business-standard.com/article/markets/india-s-silver-use-triples-in-a-decade-world-share-up-from-14-7-to-39-2-118061300779_1.html.

Liu W, et al. Impact of silver nanoparticles on human cells: effect of particle size. *Nanotoxicology.* Mar-Dec 2010; 4(1-4), 319-330.

Railean-Plugara V, et al. Antimicrobial properties of biosynthesized silver nanoparticles studied by flow cytometry and related techniques. *Electrophoresis* 2016:37(5-6):752-761.

Samberg ME, et al. Evaluation of silver nanoparticle toxicity in skin in vivo and keratinocytes in vitro. *Environmental Health Perspectives,* 1181(3), March 2010, 407-413.

Paddock HN, et al. A silver-impregnated antimicrobial dressing reduces hospital costs for pediatric burn patients. *J Pediatr Surg,* 2007 Jan;42(1): 211-3.

Acanlon E, et al. Cost-effective faster wound healing with a sustained silver-releasing foam dressing in delayed healing leg ulcers – a health-economic analysis. *Int Wound J,* 2005 Jun; 2(2):150-60.

Powell J. Silver: Our mightiest germ fighter. *Sci Digest,* 1978; Mar 57-60.

Sellman S. A Silver lining for women's health. *Total Health Magazine,* 2018, Vol. 30, No. 5, 24-26.

Silver in history:

Nowack B, et al. 120 Years of Nanosilver History: Implications for Policy Makers. *Environ Sci Technol.* 2011, 45, 4, 1177-1183.

Alexander JW. History of the medical use of silver. *Surgical Infections,* 10(3), 2009, 289-292.

Marshall CR, Killoh GB, The Bactericidal Action of Collosols of Silver and Mercury, *Brit Med J,* January 16th, 1915; 1:102-3.

Roe, AL, Collosol Argentum and its Ophthalmic Uses, *Brit Med J,* January 16th, 1915; 3:104.

Morris, M, The Therapeutic Effects of Colloidal Preparations, *Brit Med J*, May 12th, 1917; 1:617.

Silver safety:

Hill, WR, Pillsbury, MA, *Argyria: The Pharmacology of Silver,* The Williams & Wilkins Company, Baltimore, 1939; 2, 169.

Kim YS, et al. Subchronic oral toxicity of silver nanoparticles. *Part Fibre Toxicol* 7(20) (2010).

Munger MA, et al. In vivo human time-exposure study of orally dosed commercial silver nanoparticles. *Nanomedicine.* 2014 Jan;10(1):1-9.

Chang Al, et al. A case of argyria after colloidal silver ingestion. *J Cutan Pathol,* 2006 Dec; 33(12):809-11.

General antimicrobial silver effects:

Silver as a drinking-water disinfectant. World Health Organization. 2003.https://www.who.int/water_sanitation_health/dwq/chemicals/silver.pdf

Rai M, et al. Silver nanoparticles as a new generation of antimicrobials. *Biotechnol Adv*. 2009 Jan-Feb;27(1):76-83.

Revelli DA, et al. A unique Silver Sol with broad antimicrobial properties. *JSHO*, Vol. 3, April 2011.

Durán N, et al. Silver nanoparticles: A new view on mechanistic aspects on antimicrobial activity. *Nanomedicine*. 2016 Apr;12(3):789-799.

Baker C, et al. Synthesis and antibacterial properties of silver nanoparticles. J *Nanosci Nanotech*, 5 (2005) 244-249.

Jurczak F, et al. Randomized clinical trial of hydrofiber dressing with silver versus povidone-iodine gauze in the management of open surgical and traumatic wounds. *Int Wound J,* 2007 Mar; 4(1):66-76.

Roe D, et al. Antimicrobial surface functionalization of plastic catheters by silver nanoparticles. *J Antimicrobial Chemotherapy*, 61 (2008) 869-876.

Singh M, et al. Nanotechnology in Medicine and Antibacterial Effect of Silver Nanoparticles. *Dig J of Nanomaterials and Biostructures,* Vol. 3, No. 3, September 2008, 115-122.

Morones JR, et al. The Bactericidal Effect of Silver Nanoparticles, *Nanotechnol* 16, 2005, 2346 -2353.

Russell AD, Hugo WB. Antimicrobial Activity and Action of Silver, *Prog Med Chem* 31, 1994. 351 - 371.

Agnihotri S, et al. Immobilized silver nanoparticles enhance contact killing and show highest efficacy: elucidation of the mechanism of bactericidal action of silver. *Nanoscale*, 2013 (5);7328.

Roy R, et al. Ultradilute Ag-aquasols with extraordinary bactericidal properties: role of the system Ag-O-H2O. *Materials Research Innovations.* 2007:11(1), 3-18.

Rai M, et al. Silver nanoparticles as a new generation of antimicrobials. *Biotech Advances*, 27 (2009) 76-83.

Lok CN, et al. Silver nanoparticles: partial oxidation and antibacterial activities. *J Biol Inorg Chem*, 2007; 12:527-534.

Antibacterial silver effects:

Lara H, et al. Bactericidal effect of silver nanoparticles against multi-resistant bacteria. *J Microbiol Biotechnol.* 2010, 26, 615-621.

Pedersen G. Silver sol and the successful treatment of hospital acquired MRSA in human subjects with ongoing infection. *Anti-Aging Therapeutics*, Vol. 11, Chapter 35, pgs. 295-300.kk

Zhao, G, Stevens, SE, "Multiple Parameters for the Comprehensive Evaluation of the Susceptibility of *Escherichia coli* to the Silver Ion," *BioMetals*, 1998; 11:27, 28.

Dibrov P, et al. Chemiosmotic mechanism of antimicrobial activity of Ag+ in Vibrio cholera. *Antimicrobial Agents and Chemotherapy*, 46(8), Aug 2002, 2668-2680.

Lee BU, et al. Inactivation of S. epidrmidis, B. subtilis, and E. coli bacteria bioaerosols deposited on a filter utilizing airborne silver nanoparticles. *J Microbiol Biotechnol*, 18(1) (2008) 176-182.

Feng QL, et al. A mechanistic study of the antibacterial effects of silver ions om Escherichia coli and Staphylococcus aureus. *J Biomed Mat Res* 52(4) 15 Dec 2000, 662-668.

Samberg ME, et al. Antibacterial efficacy of silver nanoparticles of different sizes, surface conditions and synthesis methods. *Nanotoxicology*, 2011 Jun;5(2):244-53.

Bretana L, et al. Antibacterial efficacy of a colloidal silver complex. *Surg Forum,* 1966; 17:76-8.

Sondi I, Salopek-Sondi B. Silver nanoparticles as antimicrobial agent: a case study on E. coli as a model for Gram-negative bacteria. *Journal of Colloid and Interface Science* 275 (2004) 177-182.

Lansdown ABG. Silver I: Its Antibacterial Properties and Mechanism of Action, *J Wound Care* 11, 5, 2008, 173.

Rahim A, et al. Bactericidal and Antibiotic Synergistic Effect of Nanosilver Against Methicillin-Resistant Staphylococcus aureus. Jundishapur *Journal of Microbiology*, Vol. 8,11 e25867. 21 Nov. 2015, doi:10.5812/jjm.2586

Morones-Ramirez J, et al. Silver enhances antibiotic activity against Gram-negative bacteria. *Sci Transl Med.* 2013 Jun 19;5(190): 190ra81.

Brown MRW, Anderson RA. The Bactericidal Effect of Silver Ions on Pseudmonas aeruginosa. *J Pharm Pharmacol* 20 (Supplement), (1968) 1 - 3.

Thurmann RB, Gerba CP. The Molecular Mechanisms of Copper and Silver Ion Disinfection of Bacteria and Viruses, *Crit Rev Environ Control* 18, 295 - 315.

Swolana D, et al. The antibacterial effect of silver nanoparticles on Staphylococcus epidermidis strains with different biofilm-forming ability. *Nanomaterials,* 10 (2020) 1010; doi:10.3390/nano10051010

Bragg PD, Rainnie DJ. The effect of silver ions on the respiratory chain of *Escerichia coli. Can J Microbiol.* 1974 (20); 883-889.

Berger TJ, et al. Electrically Generated Silver Ions: Quantitative Effects on Bacterial and Mammalian Cells, *Anti Microb Agents*, 1976; 9(2): 357-8.

Siddhartha S, et al. Characterization of enhanced antibacterial effects of novel silver nanoparticles, *Nanotechnology.*18, 2007.

Lara H, et al. Silver nanoparticles are broad-spectrum bactericidal and virucidal compounds. *J of Nanobiotech.* 2011, 9:30.

Kalishwaralal K, et al. Silver nanoparticles impede the biofilm formation by *Pseudomonas aeruginosa* and *Staphylococcus epidermidis. Colloids and Surfaces B: Biointerfaces.* Elsevier, Vol. 79, 2; 2010, 340-344.

Li W, et al. The bactericidal spectrum and virucidal effects of silver nanoparticles against the pathogens in sericulture. *Open Journal of Animal Sciences*, Vol. 3, No. 3, 2013, 169-173.

Randall CP, et al. The silver cation (Ag+): antistaphylococcal activity, mode of action and resistance studies. *J Antibicrob Chemother* 2013; 68, 131-138.

Edwards-Jones V. Antibacterial and barrier effects of silver against methicillin-resistant Staphylococcus aureus. *J Wound Care,* 2006 Jul; 15(7): 285-90.

Antiviral silver effects:

Hu, R L et al. Inhibition effect of silver nanoparticles on herpes simplex virus 2. *Genetics and Molecular Research:GMR*, Vol. 13,3 7022-8. 19 Mar. 2014, doi:10.4238/2014. March.19.2

Mohammed Fayaz Λ, et al. Inactivation of microbial infectiousness by silver nanoparticles-coated condom: a new approach to inhibit HIV- and HSV-transmitted infection. *International Journal of Nanomedicine,* Vol. 7 (2012): 5007-18.

Rogers JV, et al. A preliminary assessment of silver nanoparticle inhibition of Monkeypox virus plaque formation. *Nanoscale Res Lett* 3 (2008) 129-133.

Elchiguerra JL, et al. Interaction of Silver Nanoparticles with HIV-I, *J Nanobiotechnol* 3, 2005, 6.

Thurmann RB, Gerba CP. The Molecular Mechanisms of Copper and Silver Ion Disinfection of Bacteria and Viruses, *Crit Rev Environ Control* 18, 295 - 315.

Dean, W, et al., Reduction of Viral Load in AIDS Patients with Intravenous Mild Silver Protein Three Case Reports, *Clinical Practice of Alternative Medicine*, Spring, 2001.

Lara H, et al. Silver nanoparticles are broad-spectrum bactericidal and virucidal compounds. *J of Nanobiotech*. 2011, 9:30.

Lu L, et al. Silver nanoparticles inhibit hepatitis B virus replication. *Antivir Ther*. 2008; 13(2):253-262.

Mehrbod P, et al. In vitro antiviral effect of "Nanosilver" on Influenza virus. *DARU J Pharm Sci* 17(2) (2009) 88-93.

Li W, et al. The bactericidal spectrum and virucidal effects of silver nanoparticles against the pathogens in sericulture. *Open Journal of Animal Sciences*, Vol. 3, No. 3, 2013, 169-173.

Galdiero S, et al. Silver nanoparticles as potential antiviral agents. *Molecules* 16 (2011) 8894-8918.

Fayaz AM, et al. Inactivation of microbial infectiousness by silver nanoparticles-coated condom: a new approach to inhibit HIV- and HSV-transmitted infection. *Int J Nanomed* 7 (2012) 5007-5018.

Hu RL, et al. Inhibition effect of silver nanoparticles on Herpes simplex virus 2. *Genet Mol Res*, 13(3): 7022-7028 (2014).

Speshock JL, et al. Interaction of silver nanoparticles with Tacaribe virus. J *Nanobiotech*, 8(19), 2010, 1-9.

Khandelwal, et al. Application of silver nanoparticles in viral inhibition: a new hope for antivirals. *Dig Journ Nanomater Biostructures*, 9(1), Jan-Mar 2014, 175-186.

Antiparasitic silver effects:

Pedersen G, Hedge BM. Silver Solution completely removes Malaria parasites from the blood of human subjects infected with malaria in an average of five days: A review of four randomized, multi-centred, clinical studies performed in Africa. *Indian Practioner*, 2010, Vol. 63.

Moeller WD. Malaria and TB: Implementing proven treatment and eradication methods. US Subcommittee on Africa Global Human Rights and International Operations, Committee on International Relations, House of Representatives, April 26, 2005.

Antifungal silver effects:

Berger RJ, et al. Antifungal properties of electrically generated metallic ions. *Antibicrob Agents Chemother,* 1976; 10: 856-60.

Lara H, et al. Effect of silver nanoparticles on Candida albicans biofilms: an ultrastructural study. *J Nanobiotechnol,* Vol. 13(91), 15 Dec 2015.

Kim KJ, et al. Antifungal Effect of Silver Nanoparticles on Dermatophytes. *J Microbiol Biotechnol*, 18(8), 2008, 1482-1484.

Monteiro DR, et al. Silver colloidal nanoparticles: antifungal effect against adhered cells and biofilms of Candida albicans and Candida glabrata, *Biofouling*, 27:7, 2011, 711-719.

Anwar MF, et al. Size-and shape-dependent clinical and mycological efficacy of silver nanoparticles on dandruff, *Dovepress.* 2016:11, 147-161.

Noorbakhsh F, et al. Antifungal effects of silver nanoparticles alone and with combination of antifungal drug on dermatophyte pathogen Trichophyton rubrum. *IPCBEE,* Vol. 5, 2011, 364-367.

Anti-inflammatory and systemic silver effects:

Bilstrom D. Celiac Disease Presenting with Severe Cognitive Behavioral Dysfunction in Children A Case Report. *International Journal of Psychology and Neuroscience* 6(3), 66-81.

Kailash C, et al. Effects of Nanocrystalline Silver (NPI 32101) in a Rat Model of Ulcerative Colitis. *Dig Dis Sci* 52, 2732–2742 (2007).

Baral VR, et al. Colloidal silver for lung disease in cystic fibrosis, *J R Soc Med* 2008: 101: S51–S52, 8012.

Kalishwaralal K, et al. Silver nano – a trove for retinal therapies, *J Control Release*. 2010 Jul 14;145(2);76-90.

Tian J, et al. Topical delivery of silver nanoparticles promotes wound healing. *ChemMedChem.* 2007 (2);129-136.

Silver and antibiotic effects:

Collins J, et al. Low doses of silver make bacteria more susceptible to antibiotic attack, paving the way for new therapies for drug-resistant and recurrent infections. *Wyss Institute.* [Online] June 19, 2013. [Cited: November 15, 2020.] https://wyss.harvard.edu/news/a-shot-in-the-arm-for-old-antibiotics/.

Morones-Ramirez RJ, et al. Silver enhances antibiotic activity against Gram-negative bacteria. *Science Translational Medicine,* Vol. 5, 190 (2013): 190ra81.

Iroha IR, et al. Antibacterial efficacy of colloidal silver alone and in combination with other antibiotics on isolates from wound infections, *Scien Res and Essay*. Vol. 2 (8), 338-341, 2007.

de Souza A, et al. Bactericidal activity of combinations of Silver-Water Dispersion™ with 19 antibiotics against seven microbial strains. *Current Science*, Vol. 91, No. 7, 10 Oct 2006, 926-929.

Noorbakhsh F, et al. Antifungal effects of silver nanoparticles alone and with combination of antifungal drug on dermatophyte pathogen Trichophyton rubrum. *IPCBEE*, Vol. 5, 2011, 364-367.

Anti-tumor silver effects:

Franco-Molino MA, et al. Antitumor activity of colloidal silver on MCF-7 human breast cancer cells. *J Exp & Clin Cancer Res,* 29:148, 2010.

Sriram MI, et al. Antitumor activity of silver nanoparticles in Dalton's lymphoma ascites tumor model, *Int J of Nanomed.* 2010:5, 753-762.

Singh J, et al. In-human activity and pharmacology of homemade silver nanoparticles in highly refractory metastatic head and neck squamous cell cancer. *JCO.* 2017.35.15 suppl.e17533.

Brigger I, et al. Nanoparticles in cancer therapy and diagnosis. *Advanced Drug Delivery Reviews* 54 (2002) 631-651.

Yuan YG, et al. Silver nanoparticles potentiates cytotoxicity and apoptotic potential of Camptothecin in human cervical cancer cells. *Oxidative Medicine and Cellular Longevity*, Volume 2018, Article ID 6121328, 21 pages.

Silver and the gut microbiome:

Wilding LA, et al. Repeated dose (28 day) administration of silver nanoparticles of varied size and coating does not significantly alter the indigenous murine gut microbiome. *Nanotoxicology*, 10(5), 2016, 513-520.

Williams K, et al. Effects of subchronic exposure of silver nanoparticles on intestine microbiota and gut-associated immune responses in the ileum of Sprague-Dawley rats. *Nanotoxicology*, 9:3, 279-289.

Silver and the human genome:

Genemarkers. *Gene Expression Analysis of Wounded Ex vivo Skin Cultures Treated with pH Structured Silver.* Edmonton, 2019.

Structured water:

Pollack GH. *The Fourth Phase of Water: Beyond solid liquid vapor.* Seattle WA: Erner & Sons Publishers, 2013.

Pollack GH, et al (Eds). *Water and the Cell.* Dordrecht, The Netherlands: Springer, 2006.

Cowan T. *Cancer and the New Biology of Water, 1st Ed.* White River Junction VT: Chelsea Green Publishing, 2019.

Nolte C and Betterton C. *Introduction to Structured Water with Clayton Nolte: Overview of the Health Benefits, Cost Savings and Environmental Advantages of Structured Water.* Sedona AZ: Ultimate Destiny Network, Inc., 2011.

Gann DL and Lo SY. *Double-Helix Water: Has the 200-year-old mystery of homeopathy been solved?* Las Vegas: D and Y Publishing, 2009.

Nuday C. *Water Codes : The Science of Health, Consciousness, and Enlightenment.* CA: Water Inc. 2014.

Mu SJ. *The Water Puzzle and the Hexagonal Key:Scientific Evidence of Hexagonal Water and its positive influence on health!* Coalville, UT : Uplifting Press, Inc. 2004.

Emoto M. *The True Power of Water : Healing and Discovering Ourselves.* NY : Atria Books, 2005.

Emoto M. *The Healing Power of Water.* Carlsbad, CA : Hay House, Inc. 2008.

Other interests:

Frank BL. Biomagnetic Pair Therapy and Typhoid Fever: A Pilot Study. *Medical Acupuncture.* 2017; 29 (5):308-312.

Frank BL. Acupuncture Related Techniques: What to Do When Acupuncture Isn't Enough. *Medical Acupuncture.* 2015;27(2):111-115.

Frank Bl. Regenerative Joint Therapy: Don't Replace It; Regenerate It! *Natural Awakenings/OKC.* June 2015:36-7.

Frank Bl. Stay Healthy While Travelling. *Natural Awakenings/OKC.* July 2015:34-5.

Frank BL. The Importance of Nogier's Advanced Phases for Effective Pain & Sport Medicine. *Medical Acupuncture.* 2014;26(6):326-332.

Frank BL. Medical acupuncture enhances standard wilderness care: a case study from the Inca Trail, Machu Picchu, Peru. *Wilderness & Environmental Medicine.* 1998;8(3):161-163.

Frank BL: Medical acupuncture: a model of integrated healthcare from alternative to mainstream medicine. *Colorado Medicine.* 1997; 94(7): 252-254.

Frank B. Medical Acupuncture and Wilderness Medicine: An Integrated Medical Model in Third World Settings. *The Journal of the Australian Medical Acupuncture Society*, Volume 15, No. 1, 1997.

Frank BL. Medical acupuncture in wilderness and third world settings. *Wilderness Medicine Letter.* 1997;14(2):1,6-7.

Frank BL. Medical acupuncture in wilderness medicine: an integrated medical model in third world settings. *Medical Acupuncture.* 1996;8(1):11-15.

Books of other interest:

Bilstrom D. *The Nurse Practitioners' Guide to Autoimmune Medicine: Reversing & Preventing All Autoimmunity.* Boise, ID, 2021.

Frank BL. *Travel Well, Naturally: An Essential Guide to Staying Healthy on Personal, Business or Mission Travel.* Yukon, OK: Re-Genesis Health, 2014.

Frank BL. *Auricular Medicine and Auricular Therapy: A Practical Approach.* Bloomington, IN: AuthorHouse, 2007.

Frank BL. *The Layman's Guide to Auricular Therapy.* Edmond OK : Acupuncture Medical Arts, LLC, 2007.

Auerbach PS (Ed). *Auerbach's Wilderness Medicine,* 7th Edition. Philadelphia PA: Elsevier, 2017

Li, WW. *Eat to Beat Disease: The new science of how the body can heal itself.* New York: Grand Central Publishing, 2019.

Duke JA. *The Green Pharmacy: new discoveries in herbal remedies for common diseases and conditions from the nation's foremost authority on healing herbs.* Emmaus PA: Rodale Press, 1997.

Williams LL. *Radical Medicine: Profound intervention in a profoundly toxic age.* San Francisco: International Medical Arts Publishing, 2007.

Stengler M. *The Natural Physician's Healing Therapies.* Paramus NJ: Prentice Hall, 2001.

Dinsley J. *CharcoalRemedies.com. The Complete Handbook of Medicinal Charcoal and its Applications.* Coldwater MI : Remnant Publications, 2005.

Book Chapters of other interest:

Frank BL, Schmidt S. Proliferationstherapie (Prolotherapie). In *Handbuch Nerualtherapie: Therapie mit Lokalanästhetika, 2. Auflaage.* Weinschenk S, Ed. Chapter 13.5, Pgs. 863-868. Stuttgart, Deutschland: Georg Thieme Verlag KG, 2020. (In German)

Davison K, Frank BL. Medical Ethnobotany. In *Wilderness Medicine, 7thEdition.* Auerbach PS, Ed. Chapter 68, Pgs. 1502-1528. Maryland Heights, MO: Elsevier, 2016.

Frank BL. Principles of Pain Management. In *Wilderness Medicine, 5thEdition.* Auerbach, PS, Ed. St. Louis: Mosby, 2007.

Frank BL. Principles of Pain Management. In *Wilderness Medicine, 4thEdition.* Auerbach, PS, St. Louis: Mosby, 2001.

Frank BL. Neural Therapy. *Physical Medicine & Rehabilitation Clinics of North America.* W.B. Saunders, Co. 1999;10(3):573-582.

Videos:

Medvedeva S and Anisimov V. *Water: The Great Mystery.* Accessed 2-12-21. https://www.youtube.com/watch?v=W80mHIGg9v0

Pollack G. *The Fourth Phase of Water.* Accessed 3-15-21. https://www.youtube.com/watch?v=i-T7tCMUDXU.

Pollack G. *Water, Cells, and Life.* Accessed 2-15-21. https://www.youtube.com/watch?v=p9UC0chfXcg.

Horowitz L. *What is Structured Water?* Accessed 2-15-21. https://www.youtube.com/watch?v=UkZNpeekiXs&feature=emb_lo go.

Presentations:

Frank BL. *Travel Safely from Infections.* American Naturopathic

Medical Association 2014 Annual Convention. Las Vegas, NV, 30 September 2015.

Frank BL. *Natural Health Guide for Pleasure, Business, and Mission Travel.* American Naturopathic Medical Association 2014 Annual Convention. Las Vegas, NV, 7 September 2014.

Frank BL. Course Developer and Head Instructor for American Academy of Anti-Aging and Regenerative Medicine (A4M) *Fellowship Module on Medical Acupuncture*, Fellowship Module 17 May 17-19, 2012.

Frank B. *Medical Acupuncture in Wilderness and 3rd World Settings.* Wilderness Medical Society 1997 Annual Scientific Meeting, Sun Valley, ID, August 2-8, 1997.

Frank BL. *Wilderness Medical Acupuncture.* Pan-Pacific Medical Acupuncture Forum, Gold Coast, Australia, October 14-18, 1996.

Resources for Information & Products

American Academy of Anti-Aging & Regenerative Medicine (A4M)
1801 N. Military Trail, Suite 200
Boca Raton, FL 33431
www.a4m.com
Integrative training, education and Board Certification for healthcare professionals.

American Academy of Medical Acupuncture (AAMA)
4929 Wilshire Boulevard, #428
Los Angeles, CA 90010 USA
www.medicalacupuncture.org
Membership organization for medical acupuncturists, seminars and symposia, professional journal.

American Medical College of Homeopathy
2001 W. Camelback Road, Suite 150
Phoenix, AZ 85015
www.AMCofH.org
Professional training in classical homeopathy.

MVT PRA
Micro-Vibrational Therapy - Personal Relief Assistant
2110 Pinto Lane
Las Vegas, NV
www.mvtpra.com
Natural micro-vibrational pain relief therapy units.

Natural Action Technologies Inc.
1725 W SR 89A, Suite D
Sedona, Arizona 86336
https://naturalaction.com or www.StructuredWaterProducts.com
Clayton Nolte's structured water website for products and information.

Silver Resonance, Inc.

ThankYouSilver.com, Structured Silver for consumers.

ResetCells.com, Structured Silver for Canadian consumers.

pHStructuredSilver.com Structured Silver for professionals. Register to become a professional wholesale purchaser for licensed and certified health professionals.

Notes

Notes